Touch Me Not

Lived Experiences of Patients with Leprosy

By

J.R. Berog, BSN, RN

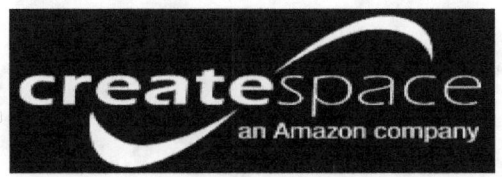
createspace
an Amazon company

Dedication

I dedicate this humble work of love to my parents who have bolstered me in terms of education, instilled the value of perseverance and brought me to where my feet stand on a pedestal today.

CONTENTS

Acknowledgment

Publishing has never been an easy journey. Writing might have already been a masterpiece which gives life to a once-empty canvass. It paints beautiful picture out of ashes and plays a good melody out of broken strings. Just like any other innately God-given talents, love prods the will and the will finds the way. It conquers all the odds in between. Publishing, however, appears like a vague countenance in a faraway vision that seems to keep the sky from kissing the sea and prevents the dream from touching the reality. It appears like a chasm that separates the heaven and earth.

Publishing a book that is anchored on a research study is for fashion, an avant-garde. It draws out the real innovation to a conventional research paper. It does not necessarily scrap out what is a cliché in the research world. Instead, it gives a symbolic representation of a culture that has been woven by Aristotle's scientific method as a way of 'seeking' for answers to human inquiries.

Now, certain people and circumstances have kept my heart melting for that desire to get this book published. The contributions of many generous and compassionate people in their different ways have invaluably made this dream a reality.

First, I would love to start relaying my word of thanks to **Clifflerey Melgarejo**, my then Grade-six teacher who was the very first person on Earth to challenge me in terms of academic performance. Because of him, I aced my scholastic undertaking.

Second, my heart shouts out loud and proud to deliver my congratulations to my co-researchers namely, **Cherebel Albano, Angeli Barrita and Stella Marie Basan.** Our sweat and tears have poured an overflowing bounty of success.

I would like to extend my deepest gratitude to **Mrs. Anna B. dela Torre, RM, RN,** for being such a smart and generous Research Mentor and for the time she has devoted in reviewing and proofreading the manuscripts.

I would also like to thank **Dr.Herminia O. Fernandez, RN, RM, MAN,** for always having been the ever supportive and dynamic Dean of the College of Nursing.

Please allow me to express my warmest gratitude to the Research

Director, **Mr. Kelly Thomas B. Tadena, RN, MAN** for his excellent guidance, care, patience and for providing me an excellent atmosphere in doing research. Indeed, he has left a remarkable opportunity for change and improvement in all facets of life and has spoiled us with his sweet and ever tender smile signifying his hope and concern. He is one of those people who have considered my idea brilliant. He has also been the podium presenter of this study in an International Conference of Research.

More importantly, I beseech to hand over my thanks to the circle of panelists during the Research Proposal and Final Oral Examination who validated, scrutinized and made professional criticisms to improve this toil namely, **Flordeliza Gagani, MAEd; Don Roel Arias, Ed. D, DA. Lit. Com.; Alex Magalona, RN, DODT; Johnny Yao, RN, DM; Alberto A. Jumao-as Jr., Ed. D. and Kelly Thomas B. Tadena, RN, MAN.** Indeed, they have greatly refurbished and polished every inch of this work to make this study successful.

Above and beyond all, my eternal gratitude goes to **Almighty God** for having bestowed in me wisdom and perseverance to manage the storm as I sail away and make this enterprise a successful one. "I can do everything through Christ who strengthens me."- Philippians 4:13

Abstract

Contracting a contagious disease such as Leprosy can be very stigmatizing for fear of the society's prejudgment suppositions. It can be a big burden and humiliating in the part of the persons affected. People with the communicable condition can suffer a lot and go through different challenges and struggles of showing one's self to the society they're living and in coping with the trials of day-to-day living.

This study aimed to understand the meaning of the lived experiences of patients diagnosed with leprosy and how do these lived experiences change their outlooks in life and influence the nature in which they live. Equally important, this study was driven by the purpose of guiding student nurses and all other young researchers in the qualitative approach of research.

This study utilized the qualitative method specifically phenomenological approach since it is a way of describing lived experiences as a phenomenon that has not been clearly described and explained. Husserlian's philosophy was used which calls for the process of bracketing. The study population comprised of 7 patients diagnosed with Hansen's Disease and undergoing treatment at Eversley Childs Sanitarium. In-depth interview was done using one- on- one interaction with the participants. Each of the recorded interview was transcribed verbatim, analysed and described using Colaizzi's method.

Fifteen cluster themes were developed which later evolved into 6 emergent themes which described the lived experience of leprosy patients. The themes depicted that the lived experience of leprosy patients is a blend of both sunny and shady proportions. They conveyed both positive and negative emotional responses. Social support has been a great aid in making a transition in their lives which were once perceived to be miserable.

The findings of this study have provided insights into the lived experience of leprosy patients. It is hoped that this study will help reduce the impact of leprosy- related stigma and become an instrument for future researchers in their fields of related studies.

Disclaimer: For book adaptation purposes and as per publisher advice, some conventional headings and chapter names were altered to facilitate readability of the general target audience.

CHAPTER I

Hansen's: the Disease of a Leper

What is it?

Leprosy (also known as Hansen's disease) is a chronic infectious disease with particular epidemiological and clinical characteristics. It is caused by the bacillus *Mycobacterium leprae,* an intracytoplasmic parasite, affecting mainly the skin and or peripheral nerves (Girao et al, 2013). Leprosy is the oldest disease known to man. The earliest written records describing true leprosy came from India around the period 600 BC (Luka, 2012).

Leprosy existed in the Philippines long before the arrival of the Spanish in the 16th century and was known locally by such terms as 'ketong' and 'cizaro'. Philippines accounts for big number of leprosy cases in Western Pacific. Citing records of the WHO, Dofitas reported that in 2011, there were 1,818 new cases in the Philippines, representing 36 percent of the cases detected in Western Pacific (The Philippine Star, 2013). The global registered prevalence of leprosy at the beginning of 2011 stood at 192,246 cases, and 228,474 new cases were detected during the year 2010 (World Health Organization, 2014).

Patients diagnosed with leprosy are constantly carrying the burden of being fetched down socially. As told by Peters et al (2013), manifestations of stigma including self-stigma, social exclusion, and discrimination, although nowadays more subtle with less ostracism, remain a reality for many people affected(Peters et al, 2013). All these social manifestations which seemingly describe leprosy patients as outcasts in the society stem to many other problems challenging health care.

The Real Pain

Contracting a contagious disease such as Leprosy can be very stigmatizing for fear of the society's prejudgment suppositions. It can be a big burden and humiliating in the part of the persons affected. People with the communicable condition can suffer a lot and go through different challenges and struggles of showing one's self to the society they're living in and in coping with the trials of day-to-day living. So the impetus of this study is the growing social stigma which leprosy patients constantly receive. Leprosy patients coming from different walks of life have all their own different stories to tell and only through obtaining individual perspective of their lived experiences will we be able to understand the meaning of those experiences. That's why this study aims to gather the different lived experiences of leprosy patients undergoing treatment at Eversley Childs Sanitarium.

Literature Says It All

Leprosy is a chronic infectious disease which if untreated, leads to progressive physical, psychological and social disabilities and dehabilitation. The associated visible deformities and disabilities have contributed to the stigma and discrimination experienced by leprosy patients, even among those who have been cured. Because of the stigma associated with the disease, patients sometimes delay seeking proper care until they develop physical deformities. The quality of life of such persons declines rapidly. Stigma toward persons affected by leprosy and their families has also adversely affected their quality of life due to its impact on their mobility, interpersonal relationships, marriage employment, leisure and social activities (Mankar et al, 2011). This poses a big social dilemma accounting to the impacts of leprosy stigma as a root of all additional sufferings of the people affected by the disease. Although stigma in consideration with its political, social and cultural contexts is poorly understood and only few studies have attempted to delve through, it remains a threat to leprosy patients.

Much effort has been brought forth and laid successful in eradicating that contagious and infectious disease. According to the World Health Organization (2014), elimination of leprosy globally was achieved in the year 2000 (i.e. a prevalence rate of leprosy less than 1 case per 10 000 persons at global level). Close to 16 million leprosy patients have been cured with MDT (Multi-Drug Therapy) over the past 20 years (WHO, 2014). However, the strife against societal issues associated with the disease is not yet fully resolved and one of which propelling through history is no other than "social stigma." According to Brakel (2003), leprosy stigma is known and referred to very widely, even to the extent that the word "leprosy" (or the local term for leprosy) is used as a curse word in some countries.

Stigma has been defined as "an attribute that is deeply discrediting," leading to a "spoiled identity". In terms of human suffering, the consequences of stigma often outweigh the burden of physical afflictions. Many people live happily with severe physical impairments, as long as they are accepted, respected, and loved by those around them and are able to function and participate meaningfully in the society in which they live (Brakel, 2003). In several studies, this happens to be true. The results of study conducted by Mankar (2011) show (a) that among the control group, 43.10% of population said that they would not like food to be served by leprosy patients, compared to 13.73% in the study group; and (b) leprosy can be seen as having psychological, socioeconomic and spiritual dimensions that progressively dehabilitate the affected persons who are not properly cared for. A study conducted by Chen et al (2005) shows that the most common reason for divorce was fear of infection; and some patients were stigmatized and experienced denial and rejection by the community members. And with another study by Kumar and Anbalagan (1983) of 225 adult leprosy patients, it was observed that 17.34%, 14.33% and 45.78% of patients experienced negative reactions from their families, spouses and society members, respectively. Out of 79 unmarried patients, 53 (67.1%) attributed leprosy as the only reason for not getting a partner for marriage. Out of 146 married patients, 34 (23.3%) were not living with their spouses; this also included 9 (6.2%) patients, deserted by their partners. Leprosy uprooted 44 (13.55%) patients from their residences, of whom 27 settled in leprosy village/settlement. The occupational status of 104 (46.22%) patients was adversely affected due to leprosy, of whom 43 became dependents and 17 beggars.

Treatment drop-out is a major challenge which deters the efforts of health care in the total eradication of the disease. Girao et al (2013) divided the causes of leprosy treatment abandonment into three categories: (a) personal (b) medical and (c) factors related to the healthcare centers. Personal factors include stigma and other social reasons, either psychological or economic, such as travel costs, loss of earnings, etc.(Girao et al, 2013). And as added by the World Health Organization (2014), the age-old stigma associated with the disease remains an obstacle to self-reporting and early treatment. The image of leprosy has to be changed at the global, national and local levels. A new environment, in which patients will not hesitate to come forward for diagnosis and treatment at any health facility, must be created (WHO, 2014). Moreover, the low adhesion is responsible for the remaining potential sources of infection, irreversible complications, incomplete cure and, additionally, may lead to resistance to multiple drugs (Girao et al, 2013).

It remains a vital role for the nurses to help upheave the adherence to treatment and to minimize other potential problems which may impede the goals of Philippines' National Leprosy Control Program (NLCP). And this can only be made possible by determining individual perspectives of the lived experiences among patients diagnosed with the disease so as to arrive at better understanding of the meanings they give to their experiences as well as to their condition. As stated in the study by Peters et al (2013), it is imperative to consider the meaning of leprosy and everyday experiences of people affected by leprosy and key persons in the community if one aims to make leprosy services more effective. To help leprosy services become more perceptive towards issues surrounding leprosy-related stigma and reduce its impact, it is necessary to understand stigma from the perspective of the people affected and their family members . However, little is written in the international literature about the experiences of people currently being treated for leprosy, those cured, or other key informants (Peters et al,2013).

The experiences of people affected by leprosy are conceptualized in diverse ways. Concepts of social exclusion, discrimination, and stigma are frequently used. In particular for the concept of stigma, several conceptual frameworks have been developed often taking Goffman's now classic work on a "spoiled identity" as point of departure. One commonly used conceptual framework is the one of Weiss. Weiss extended the Hidden Distress Model of Scambler and distinguishes six types of stigma, three from perpetrators and three from those who are stigmatized. Perpetrators exhibit accepted, endorsed and enacted stigma; the latter is often called "discrimination." Those being stigmatised exhibit anticipated (or perceived), internalised (or self-stigma), and enacted (or experienced) stigma (Peters et al, 2013).

The problems associated with leprosy stigma are soaring at its peak and becoming very obvious. As posited by Kazeem & Abegun (2011) in their study, the far-reaching and unfavourable impact of leprosy stigma leads to avoidance of healthcare services, deterioration of personal health and socio-economic status; and reduced quality and effectiveness of public health programs in controlling the disease. It also feeds upon and strengthens existing social inequalities and is manifested at all levels: individual level, in families, institutions and the wider society. Moreover, it takes place over time as a process. According to Baison and Van Den Borne, the first stage explains how certain leprosy cognitive scopes result in a range of affective responses towards the disease. The second stage involves how these affective responses contribute to social devaluation of the leprosy patient and consequently, the adoption of negative behaviours towards them (Kazeem & Abegun, 2011).

The way people interpret leprosy and its treatment influences their way of coping with the disease (Heijnders, 2004). A study by Chalise as cited by (Girao, 2013) revealed that about 86% of cases of noncompliance, have no knowledge about the disease, approximately 39% are not sure what caused the disease, and only about 14% knew that the disease is caused by a bacterium or "microorganism". Moreover, Scambler argues that people's reaction to deny or reject the diagnosis of their stigmatizing diseases could be because they regard their disease as an acute social liability. That's why, it is crucial that we determine the meanings leprosy patients give to their own disease. According to Heijnders (2004), the meaning of a disease and its treatment will affect people's coping strategies.

What do studies prove?

A study conducted by Heijnders et al(2004) concluded that explanatory models of health care workers and interviewees are different and that if we want to improve our leprosy services, more education has to be given while at the same time listening more carefully to those affected by the disease. This will give us greater insight into the way people understand their disease and its treatment and the measures we can take to prevent the discontinuation of treatment.

Another findings of the study by Abedi et al (2013) suggest

that health care professionals should pay attention not only to leprosy patients to reduce their physical and psychological but also to the community and public culture to reduce the leprosy patients suffering from social stigma.

The studies reviewed by Brakel (2003) indicate that leprosy stigma is still a global phenomenon, occurring in both endemic and non-endemic countries. The consequences of stigma affect individuals as well as the effectiveness of leprosy control activities. Despite enormous cultural diversity, the areas of life affected are remarkably similar. They include mobility, interpersonal relationships, marriage, employment, leisure activities, and attendance at social and religious functions. This suggests that development of a standard stigma scale for leprosy may be possible Data obtained with such an instrument would useful in situational analysis, advocacy work, monitoring and evaluation of interventions against stigma, and research to better understand stigma and its determinants.

A study by Peters et al (2013) shows that the diversities in people's experiences with leprosy indicate a demand for responsive leprosy services to serve the diverse needs, including services for those formally declared to be "cured."

Some studies have concluded that stigma affects many aspects of the lives of people affected by leprosy including "mobility, interpersonal relationships, marriage, employment, leisure activities, and attendance at social and religious functions (Luka, 2012).

Leprosy is considered by many as not merely a medical condition, but as a condition encompassing psychological, socioeconomic and spiritual dimensions that dehabilitate an individual progressively, unless properly cared for(Joseph& Rao , 1999).

The social and psychological effects of leprosy, as well as its highly visible debilities and sequelae have resulted in a historical stigma associated with leprosy(Smith, 1994).

CHAPTER II

The Real Impetus:

How do we unravel a leper's story?

This study aimed to understand the meaning of the lived experiences of patients diagnosed with leprosy and how do these lived experiences change their outlooks in life and influence the nature in which they live. Moreover, this study will explore their understanding of the phenomenon and the impact of which as experienced by the participants. Their life stories will help us not just in the deeper understanding of their experiences but also on how those experiences can be a surge or a call for the nurses to improve the quality of care they render to the leprosy patients and to reinforce control over social stigma.

The outcome implications and insights derived after the study will be beneficial to the following recipients:

Leprosy Patients. It's the time for their voices be heard and their lived experiences be given meaning to shape understanding of the essence they yield for the phenomenon. Their hidden feelings of suffering will be freely unleashed and brought back to consciousness of health care. Their understanding of their own condition will be enhanced and false perceptions be corrected. After the study, a significant boost of their self-esteem, self- acceptance and an improved sense of self-worth will be produced. Moreover, their emotional burden due to social stigma will be lessened and curtailed. And most importantly, this study will give highlight to the nature of the disease so as to augment their knowledge about symptom recognition and the importance of adherence and compliance to treatment specifically the multi-drug therapy.

Family and Society. This study will re-open the minds of society about the disease process by correcting their false hunches and speculation. This will help cease the society from thinking leprosy to be major societal threat. Likewise, this will encourage family members to provide psychosocial and emotional support to any members affected by the condition so as to reduce tendencies of rebuffing and neglecting them in the society. This may also help the family cope up with dilemmas and face social issues arising therefrom. Furthermore, this study will educate the family and society about the disease, early recognition and prevention.

Nurse Practitioners. The insights derived from this study will awaken nurses to become more sensitive to the leprosy patients' feelings and improve the quality of care they render so as to provide patient satisfaction. This will encourage nurses to enhance nursing management and render care holistically based on the appropriately formulated goals which are fully attuned for the physical, psychological and emotional recovery of the leper. Biases and prejudgment of the phenomenon will be prevented through self-reflection and self- awareness. They can as well help inform the public about the nature of the disease through health education.

Student Nurses. They will become more aware with the occurrence of the phenomenon. They will be able to apply and enhance therapeutic communication in dealing with these patients. Their understanding of the phenomenon will help them learn, internalize and apply to practice standard precaution in encountering leprosy-affected people with the emphasis on the concepts about mode of transmission and treatment. This study will usher them to expand and explore body of knowledge based on the subjective elements of the phenomenon and bring to practice.

Research Locale. The outcome of this study will benefit Eversley Childs Sanitarium in improving quality of health services to be rendered for these patients. The institution will have options of choice and room for improvement of treatment modalities and provision of institutional policies to regulate the safety, comfort and well –being of leprosy patients. The institution can also help lower down incidence rate or prevalence and reduce social stigma through public education and information dissemination.

Nursing Research. After the outcome of this study will be known, research will continue to develop, expand and refine body of knowledge being its ultimate goals. There will be a quest continuum for truth and never ending inquiry to arrive at origin of knowledge to satisfy human curiosity.

Future Researchers. The insights which will be obtained from this study will guide future researchers who will conduct a study in relation to this phenomenon. Future researchers will have a wide array of freedom to view the phenomenon in another and different perspectives.

Paving the Way To Reveal the Truth

It is important to narrow down the study topic and limit the scope of the study. The researcher should inform the readers about the limits or coverage of the study. The scope identifies the boundaries of the study in terms of subjects, objectives, facilities, area, time frame, and the issues to which the research is focused. The delimitation of the study is delimiting a study by geographic location, age, sex, population traits, population size, or other similar considerations. Delimitation is used to make study better and more feasible and nit just for the interest of the researcher. It also identifies the constraints or weaknesses of the study which are not within the control of the researcher (www.thesisnotes.com, 2009).

17

So this study utilized the following inclusion criteria: (a) age should be 18 years old and above (b) mentally healthy (c) must not have any hearing and speaking defects (d) can comprehend any of the following: Visayan dialect, Tagalog and English language (e) confined at Eversley Childs Sanitarium- Medical Ward (f) must not have any other communicable diseases. The number of participants would only depend on the extent of data saturation. The research locale was the Eversley Childs Sanitarium and the researchers did not intend to include leprosy patients who are at home or those who are outpatient. Only the lived experiences of the participants (together with their personal profile) were obtained and analyzed by this study. There were no specific variables or cues to be measured. Only their subjective experiences were analyzed and interpreted to produce the outcome of this research study.

CHAPTER III

Art of Unveiling Emotions: The Systematic

Fashion

This study utilized the qualitative method specifically phenomenological approach since it is a way of describing lived experiences as a phenomenon that has not been clearly described and explained. The study population comprised of the patients diagnosed with Leprosy Disease and undergoing treatment at Eversley Childs Sanitarium. Husserlian' s philosophy was utilized which calls for the process of 'bracketing.' A purposive sampling was used so that the sample population will be deliberately selected in a non-random fashion and that only the target participants were included in the research study. The sample size was dependent on the further need for information until the data saturation was reached.

Lepers: The Main Protagonist

The study population comprised of the diagnosed leprosy patients at Eversley Childs Sanitarium who were still undergoing treatment under Multi-drug therapy. There were seven participants involved in the study. They were chosen according to the following inclusion criteria: (a) age (18 years old and above) (b) mentally healthy (c) must not have any hearing and speaking defects (d) can comprehend any of the following: Visayan dialect, Tagalog and English (e) confined at Eversley Childs Sanitarium- Medical Ward (f) must not have any other communicable diseases. An informed consent was signed by the participant-to-be after the flow, mechanics, purposes, objectives, advantages (of participating in the research study) and the assurance of privacy were all vividly explained by the researchers.

The Damien Ward

Eversley Childs Sanitarium is a 500-bed hospital that is situated in Barangay Jagobiao, Mandaue City. It is a government-mandated institution tasked to administer medical care for leprosy patients. The health facility also provides medical services for non-Hansens cases.

The sanitarium covers an approximate area of 52.1387 hectares. It was built by Leonard Wood Memorial in 1982, with the most contributed funds from the late American philanthropist Eversley Childs. It was officially turned over to the Philippine government on May 30, 1930, with 540 admitted leprosy patients.

It originally operated exclusively as a leprosarium. In 1981, a new treatment, Multi-drug therapy, was introduced, which led to the decrease of a number of leprosy cases. This led to the expanded role of the institution by offering additional non-leprosy services like surgery, family medicine, pediatirics, obstetrics and gynecology.

Eversley Childs Sanitarium aims to strengthen its existing system by means of information technology or computerization and to provide the best and optimum health services to its patients. It also aspires to provide professional development among its staff and expand its existing medical facilities and manpower.

Eversley Childs Sanitarium has served as a home for most leprosy patients and for poor and ailing people. The hospital gives free medicines and proper medication to these people. The issuance of the Department of Health Department Order no. 72, s. 1994 led the hospital to become a general secondary hospital, including non-leprosy cases into their medical program(Everything Cebu, 2011).

The researchers conducted the one-on-one interview with the participants inside the ward to provide patient comfort and privacy.

Contrasting Self- Shadow and Differences

Before the data collection proper, the researchers first fostered self- awareness and determined level of knowledge, perceptions and personal propositions about the disease condition in order to avoid biased results. The researchers positioned themselves or utilized the process of 'bracketing' to isolate their pre-concieved ideas and pre- judgments which may color on how they would view or interpret a phenomenon.

The participants were asked to sign the informed consent signifying their willingness to participate in the study provided that all the mechanics, objectives and the assurance of confidentiality were thoroughly explained by the researchers in a manner understandable to them.

During the data collection, a semi-structured individual interview (one two interviewers to one participant at a time) was used with the help of a prepared guide questions. The guide questions focused on (a) giving meaning to leprosy (b) etiology (c) seeking care (d) understanding healing and cure (e) impact of leprosy. Open- ended questions were used to explore patient's lived experiences. The participants were initially asked " How do you describe yourself being a patient with leprosy?". They were given the freedom to talk freely and tell about their stories for the maximum duration of 1 hour. The conversation was recorded in an audio tape and via a video camera and the participants were informed about it to ensure credibility of the research study. At the end of each conversation, the participants were asked to listen and view at the recorded conversation for further clarification and to assure them that the information they disclosed were recorded accurately or otherwise known as known as 'member checking.'

After all the data were recorded and gathered completely, the research team performed 'peer debriefing' or cross- examination of evidence to compare, validate and make preliminary findings. The researchers used the process of "triangulation" to validate and interpret data according to different perspectives: interpretation of the tone of the voice recorded in audiotape, observation of the gestures and facial expression and and the use of words or terms.

Method of Data Analysis

The data analysis method was based on Colaizzi's (1978) approach to describe meaning of an experience and essence of a phenomenon through coding and clustering of essential themes. The following steps represents Colaizzi process for phenomenological data analysis(cited in Sanders, 2003; Speziale & Carpenter, 2007).

First, each transcript was read and re-read in order to obtain a general sense about the whole content. Second, for each transcript, significant statements that pertain to the phenomenon under study were extracted. Those statements were recorded on a separate sheet noting their pages and line numbers. Meanings were formulated from these significant statements. The formulated meanings were sorted into categories, clusters of themes, and themes. The findings of the study were integrated into an exhaustive description of the phenomenon under the study. The fundamental structure of the phenomenon was described (Shosha, 2012). Finally, validation of the findings was sought from the research participants to compare the researcher's descriptive results with their experiences or perceptions.

After the researchers have watched the recorded interviews in the camera and have listened to the researcher- participant conversation in the audio recorder for 5 times, each of the recordings were transcribed one by one and translated into English verbatim. After which, the transcripts were read and re-read and by the other researchers for further review that nothing was curtailed nor extended in the content of the recorded interview.

The method of triangulation made use of observing their emotions, facial gestures and tone of voice. These three parameters show relationship between the statements they disclosed and the meanings they subconsciously made throughout the conversation.

After all the transcripts were reviewed, each line was coded.

Significant statements were extracted and given formulated meanings. Formation of core meaning for each of the distilled significant statements requires that the researcher acknowledges the statements before and after each significant statement. Ninety- six (96) formulated meanings were clustered to form 15 themes. Each theme was identified according to the strained defining characteristics of each formulated meanings. Then the 15 identified clustered themes were then re-grouped to form emergent themes.

Extraction of Significant Statements

There were 96 significant statements distilled from the over-all statements of the participants. Choosing the significant statements was based on the objectives of the pre- guided questions which focus on: (a) giving meaning to leprosy (b) etiology (c) seeking care (d) understanding healing and cure (e) impact of leprosy.

Table 1 shows how significant statements were distilled from the transcribed statements.

Formulation of Core Meanings

The fundamental meaning or restatement of a phrase of significant statement or more commonly known as 'formulated meanings' were numerically coded with the same numeral as the corresponding significant statement. Table 2 shows the significant statements with their corresponding formulated meanings. The complete set of formulated meanings can be found at the end of the book.

Development of Formulated Meanings

SIGNIFICANT STATEMENTS	FORMULATED MEANINGS
Una, nahiubus ko's akung kaugalingun kay sa amu gikahadlukan ko. Pero karun nadawat ko na nga naa ko'y sakit. . . pero nalipay sad ko nga naa ko ani'ng hospital kay naa man diri ang naa'y sakit nga eng-ani. *(First, I got disappointed with myself because at home, I am to scare by. But now, I have accepted that I have a disease . . . but I am also happy that I am here in this hospital 'cause those who have a disease like this are also here.)* 1 P2: L1	Disappointment and acceptance are two vital stages of disease recognition and acquisition. Disappointment of one's self comes first accompanied by a lowering self- esteem due to a recognition of unpredictable disease or challenge in life. However, a good social support can aid in leading towards self- acceptance. For leprosy patients, their low self- esteem makes them think they are isolated from the rest of the world. However, when they are together alike having the same condition and living in the same environment, renewal of self- confidence will be gained. Togetherness, likeness and peer relation are all important. FM1

Nawagtang akung kahisubu sa akung kaugalingun nga nakapuyu ko diri sa Eversley. *(My disappointment is now gone since I am able to stay here at Eversley.)* 2 P2: L2	Social support boosts self-security. FM2

Development of Cluster Themes

The 92 formulated meanings corresponding to 92 significant statements were then categorized and clustered to form several sorted themes which sums up the assimilated and grouped formulated meanings with almost completely the same concept. Fifteen (15) clustered themes were made out of the categorized formulated meanings to partially describe participants' lived experiences. Table 3 illustrates how these cluster themes were derived:

FORMULATED MEANINGS	CLUSTER THEMES
*14 He has regrets though. He's of remorse because due to his physical condition, his family, friends and relatives almost forget and take him for granted completely. *36	Regrets and Depression

Unexpected disease recognition and identification entails phase of depression. A feeling of extreme sadness and denial were felt by the participant at first. ***50** The participant has regrets over some situations in the past.	
*19 He's not comfortable to live outside because the world inflicts pain and tears on his part that leads to lack of emotional security. ***70** The participant has felt the society's dread and fear about his disease. ***72** One's disease has impact on the way societal people would treat the stigmatized. ***80** The stigmatized individual is one who is not accepted and not accorded the respect, rights and regards of his peers, one who is disqualified from full social acceptance. ***81** It shows that his employer does not care about the health and welfare of his staff. The pacifying of the employees problem is	Societal fear

common place. ***85** Social inequality and motive for negative community behavior are mostly found in the fact that people fear infection by germs. The extent of acceptance of deformed patience varied significantly among those among those facing and not facing problems due to their deformity.	

Formation of Emergent Themes

The next step taken in the data analysis was to group theme clusters with commonalities to emergent themes. Fifteen (15) cluster themes were collapsed to form 6 Emergent Themes. Table 4 shows how these emergent themes were formed:

Illustration of formulated meanings and the development of cluster themes and formation of emergent themes

FORMULATED MEANINGS	CLUSTER THEMES	EMERGENT THEMES
*14 He has regrets though. He's of remorse because due to his physical condition, his family,	Regrets and Depression	"I was Vanished Away of Happiness:

friends and relatives almost forget and take him for granted completely. ***36** Unexpected disease recognition and identification entails phase of depression. A feeling of extreme sadness and denial were felt by the participant at first. ***50** The participant has regrets over some situations in the past.		Negative Emotional Response
*19 He's not comfortable to live outside because the world inflicts pain and tears on his part that leads to lack of emotional security. ***70** The participant has felt the society's dread and fear about his disease. ***72** One's disease has impact on the way societal people would treat the stigmatized. ***80** The stigmatized individual is one who is not accepted and not accorded the respect, rights and regards of his peers, one who is disqualified from full social acceptance. ***81** It shows that his employer does not care about the health and	Societal Fear	

welfare of his staff. The pacifying of the employees problem is common place. ***85** Social inequality and motive for negative community behavior are mostly found in the fact that people fear infection by germs. The extent of acceptance of deformed patience varied significantly among those among those facing and not facing problems due to their deformity.		
*20 He wants to convey to the public that leprosy has its own treatment and that it is not something to be scared of. ***41** It is known to the participant that society is afraid of socializing and dealing with him especially when it involves skin-to- skin or direct contact for fear of contracting the disease. It then eventually leads to participant's shame and low self- esteem. However he wants to inform the public that leprosy has its own treatment and once the Multi-	Societal Perception	

drug Therapy (MDT) is initiated, it would no longer be transmissible. ***53** Participant is a bit anxious of the society's perception of the disease. However, he is aware of the nature of the disease specifically its transmission. ***61** Participant manifests anxiety on how other people will react to his changes in physical appearance. ***64** Participant thinks other people have negative speculations about them after contracting the disease.		
*8 One's disease (leprosy) hinders realization of goals and dreams in life including stabilization of relationships among families, friends and relatives. ***29** The participant perceives leprosy as a physical and social barrier to attaining goals in life. Leprosy is thought to deter one's talents and potential. ***40** One's disease (Leprosy) limits one's capacity to	Hindrance	

attain goals, yearnings and dreams in life. ***57** Leprosy has been a hindrance to one's dreams and goals in life. There is a remorse over his present condition because it limits his former capability to attain those goals. ***65** Because of leprosy, he considers his dreams to be barred due to the physical and social limitation the disease brings. He undergoes the phase of bargaining. ***89** It limits or prevent them from fulfilling their normal roles in society. They may lose their economic independence as a result of losing their job, their physical independence as a result of disabilities.		

Integration of Results into An Exhaustive Description of the Phenomenon

The final step of the data analysis is the exhaustive description of the phenomena based on the integration of the cluster themes from all the participants. The exhaustive description provides comprehensive insight into the phenomenon or lived experiences of patients with Hansen's disease. Colaizzi (1978) suggests to "formulating the exhaustive description of the investigated phenomenon in as equivocal a statement of identification of its fundamental structure as possible.

CHAPTER IV

The Voices Waiting To Be Heard and Stories About

To Be Told

C ontracting a highly stigmatizing disease such as Leprosy can have effects on the leper's physical, psychological, emotional and social well- being. Thus, a study was prompted in order to fathomize the depth of those impacts greatly reflected in their lived expriences. The study focused on identifying their emotional responses to the societal stigma, the changes which the disease has brought them, and the coping strategies they utilized in order to endure the societal prejudice, fears and misconception from the outside world.

Colaizzi's methodological approach to phenomenological inquiry was used for analyzing the data in the current study. All transcriptions were read multiple times in order to acquire a feeling for them. The significant statements were extracted from participants' transcripts pertaining directly to the research phenomena. Formulated meanings were constructed from the significant statements and arranged into cluster themes which then evolved into emergent themes. The results were incorporated into a rich and exhaustive description of the lived experience.

Cluster Themes

From the formulated core meanings, 15 cluster themes were identified: regrets and depression, societal fear, societal perception, hindrance, hope, acceptance, determination to recover, internal factor, external factor, self- isolation, psychological conditioning, family, reconciliation with the society, suppport, and staying inside.

Emergent Themes

From the 93 extracted significant statements, 93 formulated meanings were made. After which, the formulated meanings were clustered together to form 15 cluster themes. The 15 cluster themes were then regrouped and categorized to form 6 emergent themes. The first 2 major themes were labelled with the actual phrase (translated into English) used by the participants while the remaining 4 emergent themes are descriptive phrases which highlighted the participants' meaning of their experience. Six (6) resultant themes emerged as follows: : "I Was Vanished Away of Happiness": Negative Emotional Response; "The Time Before Is Different, That of Now Is Better": Positive Emotional Response; Live For Good or Tramp For Life; Touch Me Not: Way of Isolation and Disconnection; A Struggle for Mammon, A Battle For One's Soul; Relationship and Society.

✕ "I Was Vanished Away of Happiness": Negative Emotional Response ✕

The participants conveyed negative emotional response wrought by regrets and acute phase of depression, societal fear coupled by society's wrong perception, and the disease itself (Leprosy) being a big hindrance to the dreams and goals in life. The lives of the participants indeed changed.

The participants expressed remorse over one's condition because of a shift in the way society views them as persons and the way they connect to the world. One of the participants fervently expressed extreme sadness:

"Nahugnu akung...nawagtangan ko'g kalipay...perminti ko maguol, di ko mudawat aning sakita...nganung gitagaan ko ani." *("My . . . imploded . . . I was vanished away of happiness. . . I was always sad . . . I couldn't accept this disease . . . why I was ever given this.")* 36 P7: L12-13

Another participant divulged feelings of remorse:

"Daghan ang pagmahay. Nagmahay ako nga nagkasakit ako. Nagmahay ko na wala na. . . maski ang pagduaw sa ako, maski pangumusta man lang, maski sa cellphone man lang. . . .maski naa'y numero ka, dili makuntak kay pawngun nila." *("Yes. There are many regrets. I regret that I got sick. I regret that there's no more . . . even visiting me. . . even just checking on me . . . even just through phone . . . though you have their number, but cannot be reached because they cancelled it.") 14 P2: L51-55*

It is known to the participants that society is afraid of socializing and dealing with them especially when it involves skin-to- skin or direct contact for fear of contracting the disease. It then eventually leads to participants' shame and low self- esteem. Being aware on the societal fear, a participant stated:

"O...pero di sila magsulti...mahadluk sila...kita nalang mauwaw...mupalit ka...magkumingking nalang kay mahadluk matakdan...kay aku naayu nako...nahumana man ko inum tambal...wa man sila kabaw makatakud ba...ako gipasabut di naman na makatakud." *("Yes . . . but they never tell ... they're afraid . . . and it's just us who get ashamed . . . when you buy . . . they only use their fingers for fear of getting transmitted . . . because I'm already cured. . .*

I have finished taking the medication . . . they don't know whether it's really transmissible. . . I let them understand that it is not contagious.") 41 P7: L29-34

Participants are anxious on how other people will react to the changes in their physical appearance:

"Kay sa karun na ingani na ka, murag kuan na kaayu sa mata sa mga tao ba murag kahadlukan na gyud ka." *("Because now that you're like this, seems like the eyes of the people denote that you really look scary.") 61 P5: L3-4*

The participants are afraid to live outside because the world inflicts pain and tears on their part that leads to lack of emotional security:

"Didtu sa gawas, muagas ang luha, sakit sa kasingkasing, makahunahuna ka pa na maghikug. Pero kaluuy sa Diyos gitabangan gyud ko na mapapas na sa akung hunahuna." *("There outside . . . tears will flow . . . painful to the heart . . . and you can even think of committing suicide. But with God's mercy, He helped me erase that from my mind.") 19 P2: L63-64*

Leprosy has become a hindrance to the realization of dreams and achievement of goals in life. The limitations incurred after the onset of the condition has led into self- frustration due to failure of attaining goals:

"Tinuod gyud. Ang akung panganduy makatabang sa akung mga ginikanan og mga igsuun. Nya natakdan ko ani. Aw, mao digyud ko makatabang nila pero katung wa pa ko'y sakit, nakatabang ko nila pero karun wa na." *("It's true.My dream was to help my parents, brothers and sisters. I got this disease and I was not able to help them anymore. But that time when I didn't have a disease yet, I helped them. But now, no longer.") 57 P6:L 23-26*

One's disease (leprosy) hinders realization of goals and dreams in life including stabilization of relationships among families, friends and relatives:

"Dakung babag sa akung panganduy sa una. Ang akung mga partidus, amigo, amiga . . . wala na. . . nilayu.." *("It's a big barrier to my dreams before. My comrades and friends . . . no more . . . they moved away.") 8 P2: L26-28*

✗ *"The Time Before Is Different, That Of Now Is Better":*

Positive Emotional Response ✗

D espite the shady side of the lepers' lived experiences, a sunny side of it propels. Positive emotional response was elicited despite all the naïve signs of discrimination and social stigma after the participants were woven by hope, courage and determination to recover and the acceptance of one's self and the nature of one's illness.

One of the participants expressed hope and optimism:

"Lahi ang kaniadtung panahun, mas nindut ang karun." *("The time before is different, that of now is better.") 16 P2: L59-60*

Leaving behind their lives in the past is one of their ways to live and start something new. They no longer want to go back to the past experiences for the second time around. They only want to move forward:

"Gikuan ko. . . giinngun ko gilimut ko na . . . naagi natu sa akua.

43

Dili naku mubalik sa akung naagian. Ingnun pa, bag-u naman ang kuan sa . . kinabuhi." *("I do . . . say I forgot it already . . it has all passed from me. I'd no longer go back to where I've gone. As they say, something is new . . . life.") 13 P2: L48-50*

The participants have a strong faith which keeps them to remain positive and hopeful in life, as revealed:

"Kani planu sa Ginoo. Pinangga ta sa Ginoo. Pero ang mawagtangan sa paglaum... ang Ginoo nagmahal natu, napay nagmahal. . .Mao dili gyud ko pawa sa paglaum sa, kay napa ang Ginoo nagmahal naku." *("This is God's plan. God loves us. But losing hope ... God loves us, somebody still loves us . . . That's why I'll never lose hope for now. ") 49 P7: L53-57*

After the felt stigma wreck one's self- image, there is a strong determination to recover soon completely especially that of the changes in physical appearance:

"O...maayu ka...malimpyu na...kanang wa nay sakit." *("Yes . . . that you recover . . . to clear away . . . free from disease.") 37 P7: L17*

"Para maayu ko...para mabalik ko ug trabahu." *("So that I'll recover ... so that I can go back to work.") 38 P7: L17-18*

✗ *Live For Good or Tramp For Life* ✗

The participants need more security in the aspects of physical, social, psychological and emotional being. Choosing to live inside for good is much better for them than going to the outside world of dread and tramp for the rest of their lives.

Disappointment and acceptance are two vital stages of disease recognition and acquisition. Disappointment of one's self comes first accompanied by a lowering self- esteem due to a recognition of unpredictable disease or challenge in life. However, a good social support can aid in leading towards self-acceptance. For leprosy patients, their low self- esteem makes them think they are isolated from the rest of the world. However, when they are together alike having the same condition and living in the same environment, renewal of self- confidence will be gained. Togetherness, likeness and peer relation are all important. Noting how one's debilitated palace turns into a haven and a paradise, one of the participants shared:

"Una, nahiubus ko's akung kaugalingun kay sa amu gikahadlukan ko. Pero karun nadawat ko na nga naa ko'y sakit. . . pero nalipay sad ko nga naa ko ani'ng hospital kay naa man diri ang naa'y sakit nga eng-ani." *("First, I get disappointed with myself because at home, I am to scare by. But now, I have accepted that I have a disease . . . but I am also happy that I am here in this hospital 'cause those who have a disease like this are also here.")* 1 P2: L1-4

Institutional (Leprosarium) support and services facilitate feeling of security and help establish self- worth. The lepers are, however, contented and feel blessed to live in a non-discriminating environment that nurtures remaining potential and state of wellbeing:

"Nawagtang akung kahisubu sa akung kaugalingun nga nakapuyu ko diri sa Eversley." *("My grief is now gone since I am able to stay here at Eversley.")* 2 P2: L4-6

"Arang- arang. Makakaon pila ka beses. . . aduna'y indut nga higdaanan. Daku'g kalipay ko. Nagpasalamat ko sa ginoo nga naari ko sa kaning ospitala." *("A little bit fine. I can eat for several times . . . has a good bed to sleep. It's my big happiness. I thank God that I am here in this hospital.") 12 P2: L45-48*

A bond between them is created through their likeness and togetherness being patients with the same condition and almost the same physical manifestations:

"Dinhi daghan kaayu tigkasi. . . tigkasi pamilya mu." *("Here, I have friends alike . . . seemingly my family.") 18 P2: L62-63*

The participants would feel comfortable to remain in the leprosarium for good than living in the outside world. As participant expressed feelings of delight:

"Karun, nalipay ko ug naa ko diri." *("Now, I'm happy that I'm here.") 30 p3: L24*   ". . . Ganahan rapud ko diri kay kung maayu naku, pwidi raku adto sa cottage ibilin. *("I like to be here also because if I get well soon, I can be left or put in the cottage.") 32 P3: L26-28*

☩ Touch Me Not: Way of Isolation and Disconnection☩

In order to cope with the social stigma, the participants need to disconnect and isolate themselves from the obvious signs of discrimination so as to keep emotional and psychological homeostasis.

Changes in physical appearance among leprosy patients influence how people look at them and in return affect their perception of self- image. So they are afraid of going out where most of their physical image is exposed and becomes a subject for societal judgment and for fear of being humiliated:

"Labi na sa . . . dili naman ka makalakaw ug layu tungud sa imung itsura. Lantawn ko gikan sa tiil ngadtu sa ulo. Sanglit wala na'y gawas-gawas diri o kung gusto man mugawas, dili na mahimu kay pakauwawan ta." *("Especially in . . . You can no longer go somewhere because of your physical appearance. I am viewed from foot up to my head. Hence, no more going out or if I want to, it can't be done because I am humiliated.") 9 P2: L28-31*

Isolating one's self from the society is one way of coping:

"Aw dili gyud. Ari nalang ko diri kay kung mugawas ko, musamut lang akung kahiubus nuon kung makabati ko sa ilang isturya." *("Never. I'd rather be here because if I'd go out, my disappointment would only worsen if ever I'd hear their words.") 31 P3: L24-26*

Another participant added:

"Magtagu nalang, magtagu nalang, diha nalang sa balay...di nalang ka mauwaw di masakitan." *("I'll just hide, stay in the house... you don't get ashamed so you don't get hurt.") 42 P7:L34-35*

Another way of coping is conditioning one's own thinking to supress and repress negatives remarks from other people.

Suppression and repression are used as coping mechanisms to forget or put into the subconscious mind those hurtful words or any unpleasant experience before. This is to lessen or stop adding burden of pain, worries and guilt inside:

"Kanang mga pamintas lagi . . . wala nalang to naku gihunahuna kay magrabihan ko sa akung sakit kung magsige ko hunahuna. Kung sakit na akung gipas-an, mas mugrabi pa." *("The teases right . . . I just don't mind about it 'cause my pain might worsen if I always think. If I already carry what is painful, it might further become worse.")* 5 P2: L19-22

Another way is the activity for diversion, to displace feelings into objects of amusement. Acceptance comes and is aided to happen when one's own anxiety is displaced and released through outside physical activity. Activities such as recreation and amusement maintain lepers' sense of physical function and emotional satisfaction. One Leper shared:

"Dawat ko nalang pinaagi sa akung gamaun na makalingaw sa ako." *("I just accepted it through the chores which amuse me.")* 6 P2: L22-23

Sometimes, the worst feeling comes after being neglected by their own families. They feel taken for granted and forgotten by their families but they repress it in their subconscious minds so as not to add emotional guilt and feelings of hopelessness. An activity for diversion becomes their way of mitigating the despair inside them and the emotional stress brought by the idea that they are forsaken not just by their families but by the society in general. One of the participants disclosed:

"Wala naman gyud ko nila bisitaha diri. Pero ako nalang na gibaliwala ka'y unsaun taman nga kung problemahun naku na, musamut kadaku akung problima mao pa'y daku ta'g problima karun. So mangita nalang ko'g kalingawan diri." *("They don't visit me here. But I just don't mind about it because there's nothing I can do, and if I think hard of it, my problem will only get worst plus I already have a big problem now. So I just find some fun here.") 22 P3: L19-13*

Another participant reaffirmed:

"Di na lang naku paminawun. Maong di ko mahiubos." *("I don't listen to them. That is why, I'm not disappointed.") 54 P6: L18-19*

☡ *A Struggle For Mammon, A Battle For One's Soul* ☡

Based on the understanding of the nature of their own disease (Leprosy), participants cited some risk factors divided into two: external (mammon) and internal factors (soul).

They believe their disease was contracted after their strenuous and messy environment in their previous occupations. Most of them attributed the cause of one's illness to inadequacy of rest and sleep and too much stress (External Factors). Wondering how they struggled for mammon, one participant shared a portion of his lived experience:

"Kanang sa pier kay elementary man lang ko, wala man ko makahuman . . . kargadur. Mao ni nga over fatigue, kulang sa vitamins, kulang sa pilaw labi na ug mag-overtime ko." *("That in the pier 'cause I was only up to elementary education, I haven't finished school . . . a loading crew. That's why I got over fatigue, deficient of Vitamins, plus inadequate rest especially if I work over time.") 7 P2:*

L23-26

Reaffirmed by another participant:

"Gikan guro ni's sa kakapoy unya kulang ug pahuway sa akung trabahu sauna." *("Maybe this comes from extreme fatigue and inadequate rest in my work before.")* 24 P3: L16-17

On the other hand, the participants tried to see relationship between one's attitudes with spiritual implication as an internal factor of developing the disease. Fighting for a pristine soul, one of the participants aired out:

"Dili ko kaingun nga tinuyu ni sa Ginoo o silut. Wala'y makahibaw kung unsa ang sinugdanan ani." *("I cannot say that this comes from God as a punishment. Nobody will know whatever the origin of this is.")* 34 P3:L29-31

Another participant clarifies the connection between being a sinner and being ill:

"Kana, kung naa man gani nabuhat, naa gyud ta'y dakung sala...naa gyud ta'y sala. Pero ang tanang tao di man maingun way maka sala, maka sala man gyud ta, maka sa, pero kaning akung masakitan, kaning mga tao muingun makatakud, mupalit ka'g tindahan, mahadluk man nimu, ikaw nala'y mulihay." *("That's if ever there's something we do, we really have big sin...we really have big sin. But all people cannot be inferred to sin not.") 44 P7: 36-41*

The participants also wonder whether their condition is a punishment:

"Pero nakaana sad ko karun, silut ba kaha ni nako? Ako nalang sad gi-atubang. Kung sumpayan pa tag kinabuhi, wa pay siguru, maka trabahu pa ta o dili na ba." *("But I can also say now, is this a punishment to me? I just faced it then. If our life would extend, maybe, we can go back to work or not.") 66 P5: L38-41*

℣ *Live and Love: The Only Way To Connect To The World* ℣

fter the onset and disease recognition, relationship to the family and the society is disturbed and altered. Some family members are starting to avoid them. Thus, they feel so forsaken.

However, lepers try to remain intact and linked with the outside world especially to their families and nearest kin, no matter how they're being forsaken and taken for granted. They still long to see their families well and in good condition:

"Oo. Sama sa nahitabu karun na bagyu, nakahinumdum gihapun ko kung unsa na ilahang pagkabutang karun. Gusto ko'ng makahibaw kung buhi pa ba sila, labi na sa akung mga uyuan didtu. Makahunahuna gihapun ko maski gidaut nila ako." *("Yes. Like what recently happened during the Typhoon Yolanda, I can still remember/think about their condition right now. I want to know whether they're still alive, especially my uncles there. I still can think about them although they once cursed me.") 4 P2: L15-19*

On the other hand, the lepers want to get in touch with the society:

". . . Malipay raman pud mi nga naa'y mubisita sa amua diri. *("We become happy if somebody visits here.") 23 P3: L13-14*

They are yearning for a humane relationship with the society:

"Makig-sabut, di man sad ko magpasakit nila'g isturya.... kuan, magsinabtanay pareha sa taw." (*"Make deal, I'll not let them feel pain through words .... understanding like a person.") 55 P6: L19-21*r text here.

CHAPTER V

Touch Me Not:

What Do We Need To Understand?

Kornhaber (2009) stated that when we want to understand what stands out for people in a given situation, phenomenological research gives voice to their experiences in singularly powerful way. The descriptions by our participants can help us understand what does the phrase " Touch Me Not" is really like. Only through such understanding that we can begin to experience some of the challenges faced by the leprosy patients.

The phenomena to be described are but great manifestations of how they perceived, coped and accepted their disease and gave meaning to it.

Fighting Against Stigma

Social stigma has become the greatest concern of leprosy patients. The stigma is brought about by the society's inadequate knowledge and misperception regarding the disease especially its mode of transmission. This societal fear as perceived by the patient as a threat to their ego, eventually leads to leper's frequent isolation from the open world.

According to Van Brakel(2012), perception of stigma and experiences of discrimination cause people to feel ashamed, and may cause them to isolate themselves from society, thus perpetuating the stereotype that leprosy is something shameful to be hidden away. It may cause anxiety, depression, isolation, problems in family relationships and friendships and reduce treatment adherence and chances of recovery. After which it starts to form a feeling of shame and low self- esteem in the part of the lepers which prompts them to isolate and depart from the outside world.

Because of stigma, role and relationship patterns among lepers are also affected. Mishra (2010) emphasized fear of rejection because of any leprosy patients conceal the disease even from their dear and near ones and willingly undergo psychological and physical suffering. No wonder, a negative emotional response was felt by the lepers because of the many factors such as (Peters, 2013) social rejection, family problems, loss of educational opportunity, fear, prejudice and ignorance of leprosy which compound the inherent psychological stress of leprosy.

Institutional Support

Quality care and services of the institution render feeling of satisfaction and security in the part of leprosy patients, owing to the social and emotional support it gives and fosters during their stay in the Leprosarium. For them, staying inside and living there for good provides a paradise of hope and an avenue for continuously developing one's remaining potentials. Their ambitions before might have not been achieved but they somehow savor a feeling of fulfillment because of the simple achievements which make them happy.

Having peers or co- lepers helps lighten the burden of being rejected by the society and families. Their likeness and togetherness as having the same condition and physical manifestations mitigate feeling of alienation and boosts self- esteem to live and cope with the odds of one's condition. The leprosarium or a leprosy home is a safe place for them where they feel less- threatened by societal prejudice and which they can say as their very own home.

A continuous effort of institution to improve health services is needed. The institution should uphold to promote a non-judgmental environment which allows the leper to grow as individual.

Concern for Family Members

The lepers have been banished away from their homes and forsaken by families but a strong desire for their acceptance remains to be the leper's wish. Family becomes one of their motivation for recovery. Rafferty (2005) emphasized that people with leprosy may lose their employment because of their disease, the disabilities associated with it and negative attitudes of employers. When this happens, they lose the means of supporting their families and often the respect of their communities, with loss of self-esteem.

The participants want to look after their families and are longing for their visit one day. The lepers remain confident about their love for their respective families no matter how hard it was to be abandoned.

Raising awareness of the early signs of leprosy among families also means that more individuals do not fear coming forward to leprosy and that acceptance of the patient is easier. Including family in the plan of care for the leprosy patients provides opportunity to help them learn, understand and accept the leper's condition and thus decrease patient's feeling of anxiety and self-discrimination.

Coping Strategy

In order to offset the pain brought by societal discrimination, participants have adopted ways of coping. The participants mostly used repression to put obvious signs of stigma in their subconscious to its lesser extent of being deeply perceived or remembered from time to time. Setting their psychological susceptibility to a minimum can help them cope and stand through all the challenges of being stigmatized. Maintaining positive outlooks aids them in the establishment of peace in one's mind.

Another strategy utilized by our participants is the self-isolation. Since lepers are already aware that public fear about their condition and the persons affected by it rises predominantly, they find a shield to bar those ill- statements, comments and prejudgments from the public. And there is no other way than self-isolation. Separating one's self from the rest of the society is a way of preventing from being stigmatized.

Level of societal awareness about the disease becomes a determinant of the potential for stigma. As concluded in the study of Nsagha (2011), results showed that lepers had the highest mean score of positive attitudes towards themselves followed by controls and contacts (P=0.00). This highlights the fact that lepers are interested in socializing with society but society on the contrary has a hostile attitude towards them because of their physical imperfections and fear of contagion.

These coping strategies arise in response to a low self-esteem. For according to **Yamaguchi et al (2013)** self-esteem is strongly related to emotional well-being and is an emotional component of personal qualities and competencies. It is generally related to how well or poorly individuals feel about themselves.

CHAPTER VI

A Rainbow After The Rain

The Conclusion

The lived experience of leprosy patients is a blend of both sunny and shady proportions. They conveyed both positive and negative emotional responses. Most of the lepers expressed and described their lived experience as a big challenge and at the same time a random circumstance in one's existence; for them, it was not planned and nobody ever wanted and anticipated of contracting it. However, a sheer of hope was laid over them. Social support has been a great aid in making a transition in their lives which were once perceived to be miserable. Rebuff from society strikes through them but it is halted because of the quality care rendered by the institution which curtails feelings of isolation and self- discrimination.

Relationships have been shattered and a connection to the outside world has been barred. Lepers are deprived of the sense of belonging to the society outside and the privilege for interpersonal linkages. However, establishing meaningful relationships with co-lepers amplifies feeling of being loved and self- worth. In the long run, their lives are shaped and given meaning through all the rolling sequence of their experience marked by the extremes of their physical, psychosocial and emotional well- being.

Implication

Knowledge of community members about the disease has a strong bearing on their attitude towards leprosy patients. People having knowledge about leprosy has more positive attitude than general public. Stigma is hard to define and measure, being a complex reality made up as it is from a mixture of belief, attitudes and behaviors. The attitude of health professionals can influence how patients and communities perceive leprosy. Educational efforts should be directed towards patients, families, and community members and health professions. Empowerment of persons with leprosy is key to success in reducing stigma and raising their self esteem. Educating the leaders and community influencers may affect their decision and allow appropriate information to filter down. Media can play a significant role in changing the image of leprosy. (Mishra, 2010)

Coded Significant Statements

Significant Statement No.	Significant Statements	Patient No.	Line No.
1	Una, nahiubus ko's akung kaugalingun kay sa amu gikahadlukan ko. Pero karun nadawat ko na nga naa ko'y sakit. . . pero nalipay sad ko nga naa ko ani'ng hospital kay naa man diri ang naa'y sakit nga eng-ani. *(First, I get disappointed with myself*	2	1-4

	because at home, I am to scare by. But now, I have accepted that I have a disease . . . but I am also happy that I am here in this hospital 'cause those who have a disease like this are also here.)		
2	Nawagtang akung kahisubu sa akung kaugalingun nga nakapuyu ko diri sa Eversley. *(My disappointment is now gone since I am able to stay here at Eversley.)*	2	4-6
3	Amigo ko wala na, nipalayu. . . Ang akung mga paryente gilayuan ko. Nagpuyu ako Sa ilaha, kasabot sila sa akung sakit, gipalayas nila ako. Imbis na tabangan ko nila, gipalayas nila ako. *(My friends moved away. . . My relatives are also moving away from me. I once stayed at their house, having understood the nature of my disease, they kicked me out.*	2	10-13

	Instead of helping me, they kicked me out of the house.)		
4	Oo. Sama sa nahitabo karun na bagyu, nakahinumdum gihapun ko kung unsa na ilahang pagkabutang karun. Gustu ko'ng makahibaw kung buhi pa ba sila, labi na sa akung mga uyuan didtu. Makahunahuna gihapun ko maski gidaut nila ako. *(Yes. Like what recently happened during the Typhoon Yolanda, I can still remember/think about their condition right now. I want to know whether they're still alive, especially my uncles there. I still can think about them although they once cursed me.)*	2	15-19
5	Kanang mga pamintas lagi . . . wala nalang to naku gihunahuna kay magrabihan ko sa akung sakit kung magsige ko hunahuna. Kung sakit na akung gipas-an, mas mugrabi pa. *(The*	2	19-22

	teases right . . . I just don't mind about it 'cause my pain might worsen if I always think. If I already carry what is painful, it might further become worse.)		
6	Dawat ko nalang pinaagi sa akung gamaun na makalingaw sa ako. *(I just accepted it through the chores which amuse me.)*	2	22-23
7	Kanang sa pier kay elementary man lang ko, wala man ko makahuman . . . kargador. Mao ni nga over fatigue, kulang sa vitamins, kulang sa pilaw labi na ug mag-overtime ko. *(That in the pier 'cause I was only up to elementary education, I haven't finished school . . . a loading crew. That's why I got over fatigue, deficient of Vitamins, plus inadequate rest especially if I work over time.)*	2	23-26
8	Dakung babag sa akung panganduy sa una. Ang akong	2	26-28

	mga partidos, amigo, amiga . . . wala na. . . nilayu.. *(It's a big barrier to my dreams before. My comrades and friends . . . no more . . . they moved away.)*		
9	Labi na sa . . . dili naman ka makalakaw ug layu tungud sa imung itsura. Lantawn ko gikan sa tiil ngadtu sa ulo. Sanglit wala na'y gawas-gawas diri o kung gusto man mugawas, dili na mahimu kay pakauwawan ta. *(Especially in . . . You can no longer go somewhere because of your physical appearance. I am viewed from foot up to my head. Hence, no more going out or if I want to, it can't be done because I am humiliated.)*	2	28-31
10	Sa wala paku nasakit, nipuyu ko sa ilaha. Maayu pa ilang pagtratar naku. *(When I wasn't yet sick, I lived with them. Their treatment to me was well that time.)*	2	32-33

| 11 | Katung nasakit naku, hibawn-an nila nga nagpacheck-up naku, ila naku giprangkahan ug wala naku'y mabuhat kay basin kunu ang akung mga apuhan matakdan sa maong sakit. Ingun sila 'Palayu diri.' *(When I got sick and they knew I went for a check-up, they eventually franked me and I just had nothing to do lest, according to them, my grandparents might get infected by the disease. They said 'Move away from here.'* | 2 | 33-37 |
| 12 | Arang- arang. Makakaon pila ka beses. . . aduna'y indut nga higdaanan. Daku'g kalipay ko. Nagpasalamat ko sa ginoo nga naari ko sa kaning ospitala. *(A little bit fine. I can eat for several times . . . has a good bed to sleep. Big happiness. I thank God that I am here in this hospital.)* | 2 | 45-48 |

13	Gikuan ko. . . giinngun ko gilimut ko na . . . naagi natu sa akua. Dili naku mubalik sa akung naagian. Ingnun pa, bag-u naman ang kuan sa . . kinabuhi. *(I do . . . say I forgot it already . . it has all passed from me. I'd no longer go back to where I've gone. As they say, something is new . . . life.)*	2	48-50
14	O. Daghan ang pagmahay. Nagmahay ako nga nagkasakit ako. Nagmahay ko na wala na. . . maski ang pagduaw sa aku, maski pangumusta man lang, maski sa cellphone man lang. . . .maski naa'y numero ka, dili makuntak kay pawngun nila. *(Yes. There are many regrets. I regret that I got sick. I regret that there's no more . . . even visiting me. . . even just checking on me . . . even just through phone . . . though you have their number, but cannot be reached*	2	51-54

	because they cancelled it.)		
15	Dili sad ko mutuu kay wala ko'y gibuhat na dautan. . . Dili sad nuon ko perpektu pero muingun ko na dili ko mutuu na gikan na sa sala namu. Kini gud among sakit . . . nakuha sa gawas, nakuha sa barkada, sa trabaho sa kahagu, labi na hugaw kaayu sa pier, kanang abog, seminto. *(I don't believe either 'cause there's nothing bad I did . . . I am not perfect but I really say I don't believe that it all came from our sins. Our disease is actually . . . gotten from outside, gotten through friends, from working with stress, especially that the pier is too nasty, those dusts and cement)*	2	55-59
16	Lahi ang kaniadtung panahun. Mas nindut ang karun. *(The time before is different. That of*	2	59-60

	today is better.)		
17	Wala na. Pero kung may pamasahe lang, ganahan ko muduaw. Pero pagpuyu didtu sa gawas, dili na gyud . . . wala na . . . *(No, I don't have. But if there's money for transportation, I want to visit. But living there outside . . . no longer . . .)*	2	60-62
18	Dinhi daghan kaayu tigkasi. . . tigkasi pamilya mu. *(Here, I have friends alike . . . seemingly my family)*	2	62-63
19	Didtu sa gawas, muagas ang luha, sakit sa kasingkasing, makahunahuna ka pa na maghikug. Pero kaluuy sa Diyos gitabangan gyud ko na mapapas na sa akung hunahuna. *(There outside . . . tears will flow . . . painful to the heart . . . and you can even think of committing suicide. But with God's mercy, He helped me erase*	2	63-66

	that from my mind.)		
20	Ayaw kahadluk na sila, kay naa man ni tambal. *(Should they not fear, for it has its treatment.)*	2	70-71
21	Sa diri, mapasalamatun kaayu ko ug kaning mga pasyente diri kay kung wala pami diri, ambut lang kung unsa'y gidangatann namu. Nagpasalamat mi diri kay inatiman man. Libre rapud mi. 'Nya usa pa pud, ang akung mga ginikanan patay napud. *(Here, I am very thankful together with the other patients here because if we're not here, I don't know what would've happened to us. We thank for being here because we are taken care of. Staying here is also free. Besides , my parents are already dead.)*	3	1-4
22	Wala naman gyud ko nila bisitaha diri. Pero ako nalang na gibaliwala ka'y unsaun	3	9-13

	taman nga kung problemahun naku na, musamut kadaku akung problima mao pa'y daku ta'g problima karun. So mangita nalang ko'g kalingawan diri. *(They don't visit me here. But I just don't mind about it because there's nothing I can do, and if I think hard of it, my problem will only get worst plus I already have a big problem today. So I just find some fun here.)*		
23	. . . Malipay raman pud mi nga naa'y mubisita sa amua diri. *(We become happy if somebody visits here.)*	3	13-14
24	Gikan guro ni's sa kakapoy unya kulang ug pahuway sa akung trabahu sauna. *(Maybe this comes from extreme fatigue and inadequate rest in my work before.)*	3	16-17
25	O, nabati pud na naku. Sakit kaayu paminawn ilang	3	17-18

	gipangsulti. *(Yes, I've also felt it. What they say really hurts.)*		
26	Maglikay sila naku ka'y tungud nagka eng-ani ko.*(They're dodging from me because I become like this.)*	3	18
27	Pero wala nalang naku gipanumbaling ilang gisulti, kay unsaun taman nga eng,ani naman gyudko. *(But I just don't pay attention to what they say because I am really like this.)*	3	19-20
28	Aw sila, bahala na sila sa ilang istorya. Dili nman lang sad naku huna- hunaun kay basi muinit atung ulo 'nya ako napud ang maalaut. *(And them, it's up to the dame luck of what they say. Anyway, I won't be thinking of that because I might lose my temper and I'm the only one who's going to be pity.)*	3	20-22
29	Aw kung wala pa gani akung sakit, nakatrabahu na unta ko karun. Sauna nga wala paku	3	22-24

	ani'ng sakita, dili ko ganahan mag-urong. *(If only I have no disease, perhaps I would have been working now. Before when I still didn't have the disease, I actually never wanted to be stagnant.)*		
30	Karun, nalipay ko ug naa ko diri. *(Now, I'm happy that I'm here.)*	3	24
31	Aw dili gyud. Ari nalang ko diri kay kung mugawas ko, musamut lang akung kahiubus nuon kung makabati ko sa ilang istorya. *(Never. I'd rather be here because if I go out, my disappointment will only worsen if ever I hear their words.)*	3	24-26
32	. . . Ganahan rapud ko diri kay kung maayu naku, pwidi raku adto sa cottage ibilin. *(I like to be here also because if I get well soon, I can be left or put in the cottage.)*	3	26-28

33	Nahibung ko kung diin ni'ng sakita pero dili ko mutuu nga gikan ko natakdan; naa ra gyud ni sa akung dugu. *(I really wonder where I got this disease but I don't believe that I come from contracting it; it's all in my blood.)*	3	28-29
34	Dili ko kaingun nga tinuyu ni sa Ginoo o silut. Wala'y makahibaw kung unsa ang sinugdanan ani. *(I cannot say that this comes from God as a punishment. Nobody will know whatever is the origin of this.)*	3	29-31
35	Aw syimpre, naa naman gyud na ang isturya. Pero dili nalang naku huna-hunaun. *(Of course, gossips will always be there. But I don't mind about that.)*	3	31-32
36	Nahugno akung...nawagtangan ko'g kalipay...perminti ko maguol, di ko mudawat aning sakita...nganung gitagaan ko	7	12-13

	ani. *(My . . . fell down . . . I was vanished away of happiness. . . I was always sad . . . I couldn't accept this disease . . . why I was ever given this.)*		
37	O...maayu ka...malimpyu na...kanang wa nay sakit. *(Yes . . . that you recover . . . to clear away . . . free from disease.)*	7	17
38	Para maayu ko...para mabalik ko ug trabaho. *(So that I'll recover ... so that I can go back to work.)*	7	17-18
39	Kay mauwaw naku sigeg gawas. *(Because I'm ashamed of always going out)*	7	21-22
40	Babag ni siya sa akung mga panganduy...unsaun man. *(This is a hindrance to my dreams . . . how can I)*	7	22
41	O...pero di sila magsulti...mahadluk sila...kita nalang mauwaw...mupalit ka...magkumingking nalang kay mahadluk matakdan...kay	7	29-34

	aku naayu naku...nahumana man ko inum tambal...wa man sila kabaw makatakud ba...ako gipasabut di naman na makatakud. *(Yes . . . but they never tell ... they're afraid . . . and it's just us who get ashamed . . . when you buy . . . they only use their fingers for fear of getting transmitted. . . because I'm already cured. . . I have finished taking the medication . . . they don't know whether it's really transmissible. . . I let them understand that's it's not contagious.)*		
42	Magtagu nalang, magtagu nalang, diha nalang sa balay...di nalang ka mauwaw di masakitan. *(I'll just hide, stay in the house... you don't get ashamed so you don't get hurt)*	7	34-35
43	Ok, nadawat ra nila. *(Okay. They accept me.)*	7	35
44	Kana, kung naa man gani	7	36-41

	nabuhat, naa gyud ta'y dakung sala...naa jud ta'y sala. Pero ang tanang tao di man maingun way maka sala, maka sala man gyud ta, maka sa, piru kaning akung masakitan, kaning mga tao muingun makatakud, mupalit ka'g tindahan, mahadluk man nimu, ikaw nala'y mulihay! *(That's if ever there's something we do, we really have big sin.. .we really have big sin. But all people cannot be inferred to sin not.)*		
45	Kanang di na balikan . . . maayu na gyud ko ba, ma wa nagyud ko'y problema. *(When no more recurrence . . . to really get well. . . to be free from all problems)*	7	45-46
46	O napa ko'y paglaum, paabutun sa gawas, o pusitibu lang paglantaw. Agwanta lang ko, kinahanglan ayuhun sa. *(Yes I still have hope to expect outside,*	7	46-50

	or I'm just positive with my outlooks. I just need to endure. It is a must to get cured.)		
47	Dawatun nalang ang sakit. *(Just have to accept the disease.)*	7	50
48	Sige pamuwaw gud, pamuwaw mao nay dugay matug, mao na balikan, niya sige paka trabaho nia napa kay samad, mao na ma grabi. *(Sleeping late, that's why it recurred plus you always work with the wound present so it worsened.)*	7	51-53
49	Kani planu sa Ginoo. Pinangga ta sa Ginoo. Pero ang mawagtangan sa paglaum... ang Ginoo nagmahal natu, napay nagmahal. . .Mao dili gyud ko pawa sa paglaum sa, 7kay napa ang ginoo nagtaak, nagmahal naku. *(This is God's plan. God loves us. But losing hope ... God loves us, somebody still loves us . . . That's why I'll never lose hope for now.)*	7	53-57

50	Sigi man sad ko, mahinawayon sad ka'y ko. Sigi man ko tan.aw tiil kuan, mao nang naapiktuhan nuon ko. *(I always did... I used to humiliate too. I always looked at somebody's feet, that's why I also got affected.)*	7	59-60
51	Sige mi'g over sa among trabaho, nya akong dugu di na gani ka supply. Di na kasukul ba. Kapuy na. Sige mi'g buntagaylabi ng dinalian. *(We go overtime in our work. Then my blood cannot even supply or can't endure. Tiresome already. We worked even until morning especially if it's urgent.)*	6	11-13
52	O, ako lang kumpletuhun akung tambal na maayu ko. *(Yes. I'll just complete my medication until I recover.)*	6	13-14
53	Ang katung wa makahibaw ba murag mahadluk, kani gyung sakita ako naman ni	6	14-17

	gipangutana sa doktor nya angay ba ning kahadlukan ning sakita. (*Those who didn't know seemed that they are afraid. This dsisease, as I asked the doctor whether this disease is something to be scared of.*)		
54	Di na lang nako paminawun. Maong di ko mahiubus.(*I don't listen to them. That is why, I'm not disappointed.*)	6	18-19
55	Makig-sabut, di man sad ko magpasakit nila'g isturya.... kuan, magsinabtanay pareha sa tao. (*Make deal, I'll not let them feel pain through words .... understanding like a person.*)	6	19-21
56	Wa ra ko masuku nila.okay ra, dawatun ra nako bisan gi diay-diay ko. Wa man gikaingun nanganduy ko matakdan ani. (*I'm not angry with them. It's ok, I'll just have to accept the fact eventough they underestimate me. I never*)	6	21-22

	wished to have this kind of disease.)		
57	Tinuod gyud. Ang akong pangandoy makatabang sa akong mga ginikanan ug mga igsuon. Nya natakdan ko ani. Aw, mao digyud ko makatabang nila pero katung wa pa ko'y sakit, nakatabang ko nila pero karun wa na. (It's true. *My dream is to help my parent, brothers and sisters. I got this disease and I was not able to help them anymore. But that time when I didn't have a disease yet, I helped them. But now, no longer.*)	6	23-26
58	Gusto nako nga maayu ko. Maka-uli nako sa amua. ...Di naman ko kaduaw nila kay striktu naman kay di na pagawsun. Makagawas mi pero kana lang dili magsakay. (*I want to feel good. I'll be able to go home..I can't visit them*	6	26-29

	anymore because they wont allow us to go out. We can go out but without riding any vehicle.)		
59	Di man ko maguol kay ug maguol ko, ang imung sakit musamut. *(I shouldn't be sad because if I do, your illness will get worse.)*	6	29-30
60	Aw, di man sa ingun gyud nga wa kay sala, di pud ko ingnun nga ngil-ad ug batasan. Makig join man sad ko. Mao nay gi ingun ako nalang dawatun bisan nainani ko wa man sad ko nagpakasa. *(I cannot say that I don't have sin and don't have that kind of bad habit. I mingled with them. I accept the fact that I have this kind of disease, I didn't mean to have sinned.)*	6	30-33
61	Kay sa karun na ingani na ka, murag kuan na kaayu sa mata sa mga taw ba murag	5	3-4

	kahadlukan na gyud ka.		
62	Sa uban gyud ba, sa pag travel, syempre tan-awon man gyud ka sa mga taw. Mao ikaw nalang mismo ang mulikay. *(Others never do, in travelling, of course people will watch you. So, you're just the one to avoid.)*	5	5-7
63	Aw oo uy. Ang nakadasig nako kay ang mga bata kay sigi man ug handum. *(Well yes. Who really encourage me are my children because they are always longing for me.)*	5	9-11
64	Aw syempre, maka-ana gyud ang mga taw nga mayra na in-ana siya kay bati siyag batasan. *(Well of course, people can really tell it's better to have this because of my bad attitude.)*	5	18-20
65	Aw oo syempre. Babag gyud kaayo hinuon. Kung tagaan pako og kinabuhi sa ginoo way siguro makatrabaho pa kog balik. Mao nakahuna ko,	5	31-35

	nganung ako paman? Kadaghan taw sa kalibutan, nganung ako pa may napilian? *(Well yes of course. It's really a hindrance.If God will still give me a life maybe I could go back to work. Thus, Im thinking, why me? Of the so many people in the world, why have I been chosen?)*		
66	Pero nakaana sad ko karun, silot ba kaha ni naku? Ako nalang sad gi-atubang. Kung sumpayan pa tag kinabuhi, wa pay siguru, maka trabaho pa ta o dili na ba. *(But I can also say now, is this a punishment to me? I just faced it then. If our life would extend, maybe, we can go back to work or not.)*	5	38-41
67	Gidawat rapud na ing-ani ko. Pero akong pamilya andam pa man mudawat. Syempre nangandoy pa gyud ko mabuhi. Nangandoy gyud maayo ko. *(I*	5	41-44

	just accepted I became like this. But my family is willing to accept. Of course I'm dreaming to live. I desperately yearn for recovery.)		
68	Sukad niatong nahibal-an sa akong uban pamilya na naa ko'y sanla, murag ila na akung gikahadlokan. Nagsugod na man ug panggawas ang mga sintomas naku atu. Nanghupung naku ug naanay nanggawas na gagmay na burut sa akong panit. Nabati naku didtu nila nga murag lainan na sila naku mupaduol mao nga ako na lang jud an gang mupalayu ug mubiya didtu sa amung lugar. *(Since after the rest of my family knew that I have Leprosy, they seemingly got scared of me. The symptoms of my illness had slowly manifested, sleep paralysis and skin pigmentation had shown*	4	4-11

	up. I felt that time that they didn't like to get nearer to me so I decided that I'd just be the one to stay away and leave our place. . .)		
69	Oo. Sauna gud nga kuyug pa mi sa akung pamilya malipayun kayu mi pero pagkasakit naku kay nausab naman ilang pagtagad. *(Yes, I and my family used to be very happy but when I got sick their treatment towards me has changed. . .)*	4	11-13
70	Nahadluk kayu sila sa akung sakit. Mahadluk kaayu sila muduol naku. *(They got really scared about my illness. They were very scared of approaching me. . .)*	4	13-14
71	Nawagtangan ko ug paglaum sa didtu pa ko sa Manila kay wala may kausaban naku didtu. Karun sa pag balhin nako diri sa Cebu murag nibalik akung pagtuo nga mayu pa ko kay	4	16-19

	dinhi man ko hingpit na naulian. *(I lost my hope for some time when I was in Manila because there were no changes in me. But now that I transferred here in Cebu my hopes seem getting back because it' s here where I've really recovered.)*		
72	Oo. Kay 1995 niuli man ko para mubisita murag lain na kayo amung mga tao didtu sa amu kay lain na ug tinagdan naku. *(Yes, the people in my place had treated me differently when I went home to visit my family in Leyte last 1995. . .)*	4	21-23
73	Nag-una ilang huna-huna. Mahadluk sila na matakdan naku. *(They were thinking ahead. They're scared that I might pass unto them my illness. . .)*	4	23-24
74	Lainan sila muduol naku. *(They don't like to get near me. . .)*	4	24-25

75	Ako na lang gidawat ang ilang pag tratar nila diri naku bisag sakit para naku. *(I just accepted how they treated me even if it's painful for me. . .)*	4	25-26
76	Nakababag ni sya sa akung pag skwela. *(It became a hindrance in my education. . .)* Tungod sa akong sakit wala ko'y nga skwela. *(Because of my illness I did not have a proper education. . .)* Ganahan unta ko mag teacher. *(I would like to become a teacher. . .)*	4	28-30
77	Ang akung giatubang karun ka yang akung sakit ni kumplekado sa akung atay. Mao gyud na akung kagul-an kung maka huna-huna ko sa akung sakit. *(What I am facing now is that my illness has complicate my liver. That's what I am really worried about*	4	33-36

	everytime I think about my illness. . .)		
78	Okay ra man naku kay sa kadugay nakung pagtambal dinhi naulian man ko sa uban nakung mga sakit . kini lang jud ang sangla ang dugay maulii.(*It's okay for me somehow I've been healed from my other illness. It's only the leprosy that took time to be cured.)*	1	5-8
79	Wala ko'y mga pagbasul.*(I don't have any regrets.)*	1	8
80	Luya na akung lawas. Mulihay na naku ang akung kaubandiri naku tungud sa akung sakit.*(I feel weak... my colleagues aviod me due to my condition.)*	1	9-10

81	Gidala ko nila sa San Lazaro para patambalan . giingnan ko sa akung amu ra mapauli na lang. Gi-tagaan ra ko sa sweldo unya gipauli sa tacloban.*(They brought me to san lazaro for treatment. My imloyer advised me to just go home. They gave me my salary and sent me back to tacloban.)*	1	14-16
82	Wala ko nila taga-i ug kwarta parapatambal. Na'y taga health center ni ingun naku na anhi diri sa cebu patambal.*(They did'nt give me money for treatment. A health worker advised me to come to Cebu for the treatment.)*	1	16-17
83	Nakig buwag man naku akung asawa tungud sa akong sakit. Wala sad ko nila bisitaha diri bisag kaisa.*(My wife broke up with me because of my illness. They never visited me her even once.)*	1	20-25

	Naa jud ko'y pagtuo na maayu ko. *(I have faiththat I will be cured.)*		
84	Wala naku'y planu na mabalik sa akung pamilya. Malipayun na man sad ko nagpuyu dinhi. *(I don't have plans of going back to my family. Anyhow I am already happy living here.)*	1	25-27
85	Mahadluk sila naku ug mulikay na sila naku. Mao nga dili na lang ko mugawas. Nilakaw ko dayun sa amung lugar para maanhi sa cebu sa pagtambal.*(they are scared and are avoiding me. That is why I don't go out in my house anymore . I left our place and come to cebu right away for treatment.)*	1	28-31

86	Malipay sad ko na nianhi . wala na may mahadluk naku dinhi kay pulus man mi parehas ug sakit.*(I am happy that I came here. No one is scared of me anymore because we are all in the same condition.)*	1	31-32
87	Dili nalang ko magpaduol nila. Ako nalangang mu pa layu nila kay basig matakdan sila. *(I don't get near from them. Ijust try to stay away so that they will not get transmitted.)*	1	35-36
88	Gidawat na lang naku na mulikay naku ang mga tao mulikay naku tungud sa akung sakit . *(I have accepted that people will avoid me because of my illness.)*	1	36-37
89	Oo, kay tungud ani wala ko naka supurta sa akung pamilya . Nawala akong trabaho.*(Yes, because of this I was not able to support my*	1	39-41

	family. I lost my job.)		
90	Naguul unta pero wala ko na lang huna-hunaa ako nalang gidawat akung sitwasyun .*(I was sad somehow but I just I didn't think about it anymore. I already accepted my situation.)* Wala ko'y kasuku sa akung pamilya. Kay ug wala pa ko ma sakit niini dili man sad mi magbuwag.*(I don't have anger to my family. If only I didn't have this illness we'll never get separated.)*	1	42-45
91	Wala man ko mawad-i ug pag-asa wala man mi'y problema sapag puyu dinhi.*(I did not lost my hope. We don'nt have problems living here.)*	1	49-50

92	Ako nalang gisalig sa Ginoo tanan. Nag-ampu na lang na tagaan ko ug taas na kinabuhi.*(I entrust everything to the lord. I just pray to have a longer life.)*	1	50-52
93	Wala sad ko maghuna-huna ana. Kini sakit jud ni naku. Dili silot naku. *(I never think about that. This is really my desease. Not my punishment.)*	1	52-53

Formulated Meanings

SIGNIFICANT STATEMENTS AND FORMULATED MEANINGS

Una, nahiubus ko's akung kaugalingun kay sa amu gikahadlukan ko. Pero karun nadawat ko na nga naa ko'y sakit. . . pero nalipay sad ko nga naa ko ani'ng hospital kay naa man diri ang naa'y sakit nga eng-ani. *(First, I get disappointed with myself because at home, I am to scare by. But now, I have accepted that I have a disease . . . but I*

Disappointment and acceptance are two vital stages of disease recognition and acquisition. Disappointment of one's self comes first accompanied by a lowering self- esteem due to a recognition of unpredictable disease or challenge in life. However, a good social support can aid in leading towards self-acceptance. For

am also happy that I am here in this hospital 'cause those who have a disease like this are also here.) 1 P2: L1-4	leprosy patients, their low self-esteem makes them think they are isolated from the rest of the world. However, when they are together alike having the same condition and living in the same environment, renewal of self-confidence will be gained. Togetherness, likeness and peer relation are all important. FM1
Nawagtang akung kahisubu sa akung kaugalingun nga nakapuyu ko diri sa Eversley. *(My disappointment is now gone since I am able to stay here at Eversley.) 2 P2: L4-6*	Social support boosts self-security. FM2
Amigo ko wala na, nipalayu. . . Ang akung mga paryente gilayuan ko. Nagpuyo ako Sa ilaha, kasabot sila sa akung sakit, gipalayas nila ako. Imbis na tabangan ko nila, gipalayas nila ako. *(My friends moved*	Low sense of self-worth and esteem is precipitated by the society's rebuff and prejudgments brought about by fear and wrong perception. It then becomes social stigma which makes the leper feel

away. . . My relatives are also moving away from me. I once stayed at their house, having understood the nature of my disease, they kicked me out. Instead of helping me, they kicked me out of the house.)3 P2: L10-13	alone, peculiar and isolated. FM3
Oo. Sama sa nahitabo karun na bagyu, nakahinumdum gihapun ko kung unsa na ilahang pagkabutang karun. Gusto ko'ng makahibaw kung buhi pa ba sila, labi na sa akung mga uyuan didtu. Makahunahuna gihapon ko maski gidaut nila ako. *(Yes. Like what recently happened during the Typhoon Yolanda, I can still remember/think about their condition right now. I want to know whether they're still alive, especially my uncles there. I still can think about them although they once*	Lepers try to remain intact and linked with the outside world especially to their families and nearest kin, no matter how they're being forsaken and taken for granted. They still long to see their families well and in good condition. FM4

cursed me.) 4 P2: L15-19	
Kanang mga pamintas lagi . . . wala nalang to naku gihunahuna kay magrabihan ko sa akung sakit kung magsige ko hunahuna. Kung sakit na akung gipas-an, mas mugrabi pa. *(The teases right . . . I just don't mind about it 'cause my pain might worsen if I always think. If I already carry what is painful, it might further become worse.)5 P2: L19-20*	Suppression and repression are used as coping mechanisms to forget or put into the subconscious mind those hurtful words or any unpleasant experience before. This is to lessen or stop adding burden of pain, worries and guilt inside. In the long run,it is also related to socio-economic status. FM5
Dawat ko nalang pinaagi sa akung gamaun na makalingaw sa ako. *(I just accepted it through the chores which amuse me.)6 P2: L22-23*	Acceptance comes and is aided to happen when one's own anxiety is displaced and released through outside physical activity. Activities such as recreation and amusement maintains lepers' sense of physical function and emotional satisfaction. FM6
Kanang sa pier kay elementary man lang ko, wala	He conceives leprosy to be caused by physiologic

man ko makahuman . . . kargadur. Mao ni nga over fatigue, kulang sa vitamins, kulang sa pilaw labi na ug mag-overtime ko. *(That in the pier 'cause I was only up to elementary education, I haven't finished school . . . a loading crew. That's why I got over fatigue, deficient of Vitamins, plus inadequate rest especially if I work over time.)7 P2: L23-26*	insufficiencies and lack of optimum health habits related to work and stress of his previous job. Specifically, he attributed inadequate rest as one of the major determinants of developing leprosy. FM7
Dakung babag sa akung panganduy sa una. Ang akung mga partidus, amigo, amiga . . . wala na. . . nilayu.. *(It's a big barrier to my dreams before. My comrades and friends . . . no more . . . they moved away.)8 P2: L26-28*	One's disease (leprosy) hinders realization of goals and dreams in life including stabilization of relationships among families, friends and relatives. FM8
Labi na sa . . . dili naman ka makalakaw ug layu tungod sa imung itsura. Lantawn ko gikan sa tiil ngadtu sa ulo.	Changes in physical appearance among leprosy patients influence how people look at them and in return

Sanglit wala na'y gawas-gawas diri o kung gusto man mugawas, dili na mahimu kay pakauwawan ta. *(Especially in . . . You can no longer go somewhere because of your physical appearance. I am viewed from foot up to my head. Hence, no more going out or if I want to, it can't be done because I am humiliated.)9 P2: L28-31*	affect their perception of self-image. So they are afraid of going out where most of their physical image is exposed and becomes a subject for societal judgment and for fear of being humiliated. FM9
Sa wala paku nasakit, nipuyu ko sa ilaha. Maayu pa ilang pagtratar naku. *(When I wasn't yet sick, I lived with them. Their treatment to me was well that time.)10 P2: L32-33*	Relationship changes and the role- pattern is disturbed between the family members and the patient after recognition of disease condition. FM10
Katung nasakit naku, hibawn-an nila nga nagpacheck-up naku, ila naku giprangkahan ug wala naku'y mabuhat kay basin kunu ang akung mga apuhan matakdan sa maong sakit. Ingun sila 'Palayu diri.'	He was forced to move out of the house for fear of transmitting the disease to other family members and infecting those whom he loves. FM11

(When I got sick and they knew I went for a check-up, they eventually franked me and I just had nothing to do lest, according to them, my grandparents might get infected by the disease. They said 'Move away from here.'11 P12: L33-37	
Arang- arang. Makakaon pila ka beses. . . aduna'y indot nga higdaanan. Daku'g kalipay ko. Nagpasalamat ko sa ginoo nga naari ko sa kaning ospitala. *(A little bit fine. I can eat for several times . . . has a good bed to sleep. Big happiness. I thank God that I am here in this hospital.) 12 P2: L45-48*	Institutional (Leprosarium) support and services facilitate feeling of security and help establish self- worth. The lepers are, however, contented and feel blessed to live in a non-discriminating environment that nurtures remaining potential and state of wellbeing. FM12
Gikuan ko. . . giinngun ko gilimut ko na . . . naagi natu sa akua. Dili naku mubalik sa akung naagian. Ingnun pa, bag-u naman ang kuan sa . .	Leaving behind their lives in the past is one of their ways to live and start something new. They no longer want to go back to the past experiences

kinabuhi. *(I do . . . say I forgot it already . . it has all passed from me. I'd no longer go back to where I've gone. As they say, something is new . . . life.)13 P2: L48-50*	for the second time around. They only want to move forward. FM13
O. Daghan ang pagmahay. Nagmahay ako nga nagkasakit ako. Nagmahay ko na wala na. . . maski ang pagduaw sa aku, maski pangumusta man lang, maski sa cellphone man lang. . . .maski naa'y numero ka, dili makuntak kay pawngun nila. *(Yes. There are many regrets. I regret that I got sick. I regret that there's no more . . . even visiting me. . . even just checking on me . . . even just through phone . . . though you have their number, but cannot be reached because they cancelled it.) 14 P2: L51-54*	He has regrets though. He's of remorse because due to his physical condition, his family, friends and relatives almost forget and take him for granted completely. FM14
Dili sad ko mutuu kay wala	He perceived his disease to be

ko'y gibuhat na dautan. . . Dili sad nuon ko perpektu pero muingun ko na dili ko mutuu na gikan na sa sala namu. Kini gud amung sakit . . . nakuha sa gawas, nakuha sa barkada, sa trabaho sa kahagu, labi na hugaw kaayu sa pier, kanang abog, seminto. *(I don't believe either 'cause there's nothing bad I did . . . I am not perfect but I really say I don't believe that it all came from our sins. Our disease is actually . . . gotten from outside, gotten through friends, from working with stress, especially that the pier is too nasty, those dusts and cement)15 P2: L55-59*	caused by external factors such as occupation, inadequate rest and companion. He does not believe that it comes from internal factors such as a person's attitude and character attributed to one's own personality in general. FM15
Lahi ang kaniadtung panahun. Mas nindut ang karun. *(The time before is different. That of now is better.)16 P2: L59-60*	He views past as something different. He's a lot more hopeful with the present. FM16
Wala na. Pero kung may	He's willing to go home if

pamasahe lang, ganahan ko muduaw. Pero pagpuyu didtu sa gawas, dili na gyud . . . wala na . . . *(No, I don't have. But if there's money for transportation, I want to visit. But living there outside . . . no longer . . .) 17 P2: L60-62*	there's any chance, but is only limited to visiting his family and not to living there forever. He'd prefer and is more comfortable to stay inside the Leprosarium for good. FM17
Dinhi daghan kaayu tigkasi. . . tigkasi pamilya mu. *(Here, I have friends alike . . . seemingly my family)18 P2: L62-63*	He assumes his co-lepers to be his peers whom he also considers his family. A bond between them is created through their likeness and togetherness being patients with the same condition and almost the same physical manifestations. FM18
Didtu sa gawas, muagas ang luha, sakit sa kasingkasing, makahunahuna ka pa na maghikug. Pero kaluuy sa Diyos gitabangan gyud ko na mapapas na sa akung hunahuna. *(There outside . . . tears will flow . . . painful to the*	He's not comfortable to live outside because the world inflicts pain and tears on his part that leads to lack of emotional security. FM19

heart . . . and you can even think of committing suicide. But with God's mercy, He helped me erase that from my mind.) 19 P2: L63-66	
Ayaw kahadluk na sila, kay naa man ni tambal. *(Should they not fear, for it has its treatment.)20 P2: L70-71*	He wants to convey to the public that leprosy has its own treatment and that it is not something to be scared of. FM20
Sa diri, mapasalamatun kaayu ko ug kaning mga pasyente diri kay kung wala pami diri, ambut lang kung unsa'y gidangatann namu. Nagpasalamat mi diri kay inatiman man. Libre rapud mi. 'Nya usa pa pud, ang akung mga ginikanan patay napud. *(Here, I am very thankful together with the other patients here because if we're not here, I don't know what would've happened to us. We thank for being here because*	The patients feel secured inside the leprosarium with the services and care rendered by the institution. The leprosarium becomes their safe haven to live peacefully. They thought, had they not been brought there, living in the outside world would be more difficult. FM21

we are taken care of. Staying here is also free. Besides , my parents are already dead.) 21 P3: L1-4	
Wala naman gyud ko nila bisitaha diri. Pero ako nalang na gibaliwala ka'y unsaun taman nga kung problemahun naku na, musamut kadaku akung problima mao pa'y daku ta'g problima karun. So mangita nalang ko'g kalingawan diri. *(They don't visit me here. But I just don't mind about it because there's nothing I can do, and if I think hard of it, my problem will only get worst plus I already have a big problem today. So I just find some fun here.)22 P3: L9-13*	They feel taken for granted and forgotten by their families but they repress it in their subconscious minds so as not to add emotional guilt and feelings of hopelessness. An activity for diversion becomes their way of mitigating the despair inside them and the emotional stress brought by the idea that they're forsaken not just by their families but by the society in general. FM22
. . . Malipay raman pud mi nga naa'y mubisita sa amua diri. *(We become happy if somebody*	They are yearning to be loved and to feel the sense of belongingness, that somehow

visits here.)23 P3: L13-14	they are given worth and importance by the society and the world outside. FM23
Gikan guro ni's sa kakapoy unya kulang ug pahuway sa akung trabahu sauna. *(Maybe this comes from extreme fatigue and inadequate rest in my work before.)24 P3: L16-17*	He attributed the predisposing factors of his disease to include inadequate rest due to his previous job. FM24
O, nabati pud na naku. Sakit kaayu paminawn ilang gipangsulti. *(Yes, I've also felt it. What they say really hurts.)* 25 P3: L17-18	Discrimination is common. It tortures them verbally. FM25
Maglikay sila naku ka'y tungud nagka eng-ani ko.*(They're dodging from me because I become like this.)* 26 P3: L18	He thinks his disease becomes something to be scared of that's why others would avoid him. FM26
Pero wala nalang naku gipanumbaling ilang gisulti, kay unsaun taman nga eng,ani naman gyudko. *(But I just don't pay attention to what they say because I am really*	He has accepted himself and his disease so he shrugs at other people's prejudice. FM 27

like this.)27 P3: L19-20	
Aw sila, bahala na sila sa ilang isturya. Dili nman lang sad naku huna- hunaun kay basi muinit atung ulo 'nya ako napud ang maalaut. *(And them, it's up to the dame luck of what they say. Anyway, I won't be thinking of that because I might lose my temper and I'm the only one who's going to be pity.)28 P3: L20-22*	He is indifferent to what others might say about his disease/ condition. Minding about their statements might only precipitate self- pity and elicit both emotional and psychological jeopardy. FM28
Aw kung wala pa gani akung sakit, nakatrabahu na unta ko karun. Sauna nga wala paku ani'ng sakita, dili ko ganahan mag-urong. *(If only I have no disease, perhaps I would have been working now. Before when I still didn't have the disease, I actually never wanted to be stagnant.) 29 P3: L22-24*	The participant perceives leprosy as a physical and social barrier to attaining goals in life. Leprosy is thought to deter one's talents and potential. FM29
Karun, nalipay ko ug naa ko diri. *(Now, I'm happy that I'm*	He is happy to be in the Leprosarium. FM30

here.) 30 p3: L24	
Aw dili gyud. Ari nalang ko diri kay kung mugawas ko, musamut lang akung kahiubos nuon kung makabati ko sa ilang isturya. *(Never. I'd rather be here because if I go out, my disappointment will only worsen if ever I hear their words.)31 P3: L24-26*	He prefers not to go outside to avoid encountering obvious signs of discrimination. FM31
. . . Ganahan rapud ko diri kay kung maayu naku, pwidi raku adtu sa cottage ibilin. *(I like to be here also because if I get well soon, I can be left or put in the cottage.) 32 P3: L26-28*	He likes to stay inside and if ever he gets well, he'd prefer to stay in the cottage. than living in the outside world. He feels more safe and secured when living inside the leprosarium. FM32
Nahibung ko kung diin ni'ng sakita pero dili ko mutuu nga gikan ko natakdan; naa ra gyud ni sa akung dugo. *(I really wonder where I got this disease but I don't believe that I come from contracting it; it's all in my blood.)33 P3: L28-29*	He lacks enough knowledge about the aetiology of the disease. FM33

Dili ko kaingun nga tinuyu ni sa Ginoo o silut. Wala'y makahibaw kung unsa ang sinugdanan ani. *(I cannot say that this comes from God as a punishment. Nobody will know whatever is the origin of this.)34 P3:L29-31*	Does not attribute one's disease as God's plan. He is not certain with what really causes the disease.FM34
Aw syimpre, naa naman gyud na ang isturya. Pero dili nalang naku huna-hunaun. *(Of course, gossips will always be there. But I don't mind about that.)35 P3: L31-32*	Aware of the society's prejudice and discrimination but is willing to pay no attention to them because of self- acceptance. FM35
Nahugnu akung...nawagtangan ko'g kalipay...perminti ko maguol, di ko mudawat aning sakita...nganung gitagaan ko ani. *(My . . . fell down . . . I was vanished away of happiness. . . I was always sad . . . I couldn't accept this disease . . . why I*	Unexpected disease recognition and identification entails phase of depression. A feeling of extreme sadness and denial were felt by the participant at first. FM36

was ever given this.) 36 P7: L12-13	
O...maayu ka...malimpyu na...kanang wa nay sakit. *(Yes. . . that you recover . . . to clear away . . . free from disease.)* 37 P7: L17	There is a strong determination to recover soon completely especially that of the changes in physical appearance. FM37
Para maayu ko...para mabalik ko ug trabaho. *(So that I'll recover ... so that I can go back to work.)*38 P7: L17-18	One of the main reasons of wishing to get cured is about restoring back their previous functions for productivity. FM38
Kay mauwaw naku sigeg gawas. *(Because I'm ashamed of always going out)*39 P7: L21-22	Exposure to the society is avoided due to perception of shame brought about by one's disturbed self- image. FM39
Babag ni siya sa akung mga panganduy...unsaon man. *(This is a hindrance to my dreams . . . how can I)* 40 P7: L22	One's disease (Leprosy) limits one's capacity to attain goals, yearnings and dreams in life. FM40
O...pero di sila magsulti...mahadluk sila...kita nalang mauwaw...mupalit ka...magkumingking nalang	It is known to the participant that society is afraid of socializing and dealing with him especially when it

kay mahadluk matakdan...kay aku naayu naku...nahumana man ko inum tambal...wa man sila kabaw makatakud ba...ako gipasabut di naman na makatakud. *(Yes . . . but they never tell ... they're afraid . . . and it's just us who get ashamed . . . when you buy . . . they only use their fingers for fear of getting transmitted . . . because I'm already cured. . . I have finished taking the medication . . . they don't know whether it's really transmissible. . . I let them understand that's it is not contagious.) 41 P7: L29-34*	involves skin-to- skin or direct contact for fear of contracting the disease. It then eventually leads to participant's shame and low self- esteem. However he wants to inform the public that leprosy has its own treatment and once the Multi-drug Therapy (MDT) is initiated, it would no longer be transmissible. FM41
Magtagu nalang, magtagu nalang, diha nalang sa balay...di nalang ka mauwaw di masakitan. *(I'll just hide, stay in the house... you don't get ashamed so you don't get hurt) 42 P7:L34-35*	Hiding from the society is their way of controlling or avoiding from getting hurt. FM42

Ok, nadawat ra nila. *(Okay. They accept me.) 43 P7: L35*	There is acceptance by the family somehow. FM43
Kana, kung naa man gani nabuhat, naa gyud ta'y dakung sala...naa jud ta'y sala. Pero ang tanang tao di man maingun way maka sala, maka sala man gyud ta, maka sa, piro kaning akung masakitan, kaning mga tao muingun makatakud, mupalit ka'g tindahan, mahadluk man nimu, ikaw nala'y mulihay! *(That's if ever there's something we do, we really have big sin.. .we really have big sin. But all people cannot be inferred to sin not.) 44 P7: L36-41*	Does not attribute one's disease to be God's plan. Each one of us has our own share of sins. Fm44
Kanang di na balikan . . . maayu na gyud ko ba, ma wa nagyud ko'y problema. *(When no more recurrence . . . to really get well. . . to be free from all problems)45 P7: L45-*	There is a strong desire to get completely cured or healed. FM45

46	
O napa ko'y paglaum, paabutun sa gawas, o pusitibu lang paglantaw. Agwanta lang ko, kinahanglan ayuhun sa. *(Yes I still have hope to expect outside, or I'm just positive with my outlooks. I just need to endure. It is a must to get cured.) 46 P7: L46-50*	Hopeful and positive outlooks. All it takes to recover is patience and endurance. FM46
Dawatun nalang ang sakit. *(Just have to accept the disease.) 47 P7: L50*	There is a need for acceptance of one's condition. FM47
Sige pamuwaw gud, pamuwaw mao nay dugay matug, mao na balikan, niya sige paka trabaho nia napa kay samad, mao na ma grabi. *(Sleeping late, that's why it recurred plus you always work with the wound present so it worsened.) 48 P7: L51-53*	For him , leprosy is caused by external factors such as work- related stress and inadequate rest. FM 48
Kani plano sa Ginoo. Pinangga ta sa Ginoo. Pero ang mawagtangan sa paglaum…	Has a strong faith which keeps him to remain positive and hopeful in life. FM 49

ang Ginoo nagmahal natu, napay nagmahal. . .Mao dili gyud ko pawa sa paglaum sa, 7kay napa ang ginoo nagtaak, nagmahal naku. *(This is God's plan. God loves us. But losing hope ... God loves us, somebody still loves us . . . That's why I'll never lose hope for now.)* 49PZ: L53-57	
Sigi man sad ko, mahinawayon sad ka'y ko. Sigi man ko tan.aw tiil kuan, mao nang naapiktuhan nuon ko. *(I always did... I used to humiliate too. I always looked at somebody's feet, that's why I also got affected.)* 50 P7: L59-60	The participant has regrets over some situations in the past. FM50
Sige mi'g over sa among trabaho, nya akong dugo di na gani ka supply. Di na kasukol ba. Kapoy na. Sige mi'g buntagaylabi ng dinalian. *(We go overtime in our work. Then*	One of the perceived reasons for having leprosy is work-related factor. FM 51

my blood cannot even supply or can't endure. Tiresome already. We worked even until morning especially if it's urgent.)51 P6: L11-13	
O, ako lang kumpletuhun akong tambal na maayu ko. (*Yes. I'll just complete my medication until I recover.*) 52 P6: L13-14	Participant is aware of the nature of the Multi- Drug Therapy (MDT). FM52
Ang katong wa makahibaw ba murag mahadlok, kani gyung sakita ako naman ni gipangutana sa doktor nya angay ba ning kahadlukan ning sakita. (*Those who didn't know seemed that they are afraid. This dsisease, as I asked the doctor whether this disease is something to be scared of.*) 53 P6: L14-17	Participant is a bit anxious of the society's perception of the disease. However, he is aware of the nature of the disease specifically its transmission. FM53
Di na lang naku paminawun. Maong di ko mahiubus.(*I don't listen to them. That is why, I'm not disappointed.*)54 P6: L18-	Tolerating what others say is a coping strategy to avoid disappointment. FM54

19	
Makig-sabut, di man sad ko magpasakit nila'g isturya.... kuan, magsinabtanay pareha sa taw. (*Make deal, I'll not let them feel pain through words .... understanding like a person.)55 P6: L19-21*	Participant wants to reconcile with the society and foster humane relationship. FM55
Wa ra ko masuko nila. Okay ra, dawatun ra naku bisan gi diay-diay ko. Wa man gikaingon nanganduy ko matakdan ani. *(I'm not angry with them. It's ok, I'll just have to accept the fact even though they underestimate me. I never wished to have this kind of disease.) 56 P6: L21-22*	The participant is willing to tolerate discrimination from the society because he perceived leprosy as uncontrollable, something he never wished to have and whose reason of having is not known to him. FM56
Tinuod gyud. Ang akong panganduy makatabang sa akong mga ginikanan ug mga igsuon. Nya natakdan ko ani. Aw, mao digyud ko makatabang nila pero katong wa pa ko'y sakit, nakatabang	Leprosy has been a hindrance to one's dreams and goals in life. There is a remorse over his present condition because it limits his former capability to attain those goals. FM 57

ko nila pero karun wa na. *(It's true.My dream is to help my parent, brothers and sisters. I got this disease and I was not able to help them anymore. But that time when I didn't have a disease yet, I helped them. But now, no longer.)57 P6:L 23-26*	
Gusto nako nga maayu ko. Maka-uli nako sa amua. ...Di naman ko kaduaw nila kay striktu naman kay di na pagawson. Makagawas mi pero kana lang dili magsakay. *(I want to feel good. I'll be able to go home..I can't visit them anymore because they won' t allow us to go out. We can go out but without riding any vehicle.) 58 P6: L26-29*	To get cured and recover soon are two yearnings which the participant wishes. Moreover, he still misses his family so much and is longing to see them someday.FM58
Di man ko maguol kay ug maguol ko, ang imung sakit musamut. *(I shouldn't be sad because if I do, your illness will get worse.) 59 P6: L29-30*	He relates psychological mind set as a determinant to one's own physical condition. Thinking positively, for him, helps avoid his disease from

	getting worse. FM59
Aw, di man sa ingon gyud nga wa kay sala, di pud ko ingnun nga ngil-ad ug batasan. Makig join man sad ko. Mao nay gi ingun ako nalang dawatun bisan nainani ko wa man sad ko nagpakasa. (*I cannot say that I don't have sin and don't have that kind of bad habit. I mingled with them. I accept the fact that I have this kind of disease, I didn't mean to have sinned.*) 60 P6: L30-33	The participant does not perceive the relationship between attitude and one's own illness. FM60
Kay sa karun na ingani na ka, murag kuan na kaayu sa mata sa mga taw ba murag kahadlukan na gyud ka. (*Because now that you're like this, seems like the eyes of the people denote that you really look scary*) 61 P5: L3-4	Participant manifests anxiety on how other people will react to his changes in physical appearance. FM61
Sa uban gyud ba, sa pag travel, syempre tan-awon man gyud ka sa mga taw. Mao ikaw	Because of awareness on societal stigma, lepers tend to hide from the society in order

nalang mismo ang mulikay. *(Others never do, in travelling, of course people will watch you. So, you're just the one to avoid.) 62 P5: L5-7*	to isolate themselves in a way they are less- threatened by discrimination. FM62
Aw oo uy. Ang nakadasig nako kay ang mga bata kay sigi man ug handom. *(Well yes. Who really encourage me are my children because they are always longing for me.) 63 P5: L9-11*	For him, his family becomes his motivation to recover soon. FM63
Aw syempre, maka-ana gyud ang mga taw nga mayra na in-ana siya kay bati siyag batasan. *(Well of course, people can really tell it's better to have this because of my bad attitude.) 64 P5: L18-20*	Participant thinks other people have negative speculations about them after contracting the disease. FM64
Aw oo syempre. Babag gyud kaayu hinuon. Kung tagaan pako ug kinabuhi sa ginoo way siguro makatrabaho pa ko'g balik. Mao nakahuna ko, nganung ako paman?	Because of leprosy, he considers his dreams to be barred due to the physical and social limitation the disease brings. He undergoes the phase of bargaining. FM65

Kadaghan taw sa kalibutan, nganong ako pa may napilian? *(Well yes of course. It's really a hindrance.If God will still give me a life maybe I could go back to work. Thus, Im thinking, why me? Of the so many people in the world, why have I been chosen?)*65 P5 : L31-35	
Pero nakaana sad ko karon, silot ba kaha ni nako? Ako nalang sad gi-atubang. Kung sumpayan pa tag kinabuhi, wa pay siguro, maka trabaho pa ta o dili na ba. *(But I can also say now, is this a punishment to me? I just faced it then. If our life would extend, maybe, we can go back to work or not.)* 66 P5: L38-41	The participant also wonders whether his condition is a punishment. Accepting it becomes his coping strategy to move forward. Nonetheless, he is uncertain whether he can still go back to his normal life or not after overcoming the challenge wrought by his condition. FM66
Gidawat rapud na ing-ani ko. Pero akung pamilya andam pa man mudawat. Syempre nangandoy pa gyud ko mabuhi. Nangandoy gyud	Family. They are the sole motivation for the patient to recover. He becomes hopeful because of them. FM67

maayo ko. (*I just accepted I became like this. But my family is willing to accept. Of course I'm dreaming to live. I desperately yearn for recovery.)67 P5: L41-44*	
Sukad niatung nahibal-an sa akong uban pamilya na naa ko'y sanla, murag ila na akung gikahadlokan. Nagsugod na man ug panggawas ang mga sintumas naku ato. Nanghupung naku ug naanay nanggawas na gagmay na burot sa akong panit. Nabati naku didtu nila nga murag lainan na sila naku mupaduol mao nga ako na lang jud an gang mupalayu ug mubiya didtu sa amung lugar. *(Since after the rest of my family knew that I have Leprosy, they seemingly got scared of me. The symptoms of my illness had slowly manifested, sleep*	The way other people view his condition has also changed the way he perceives his self-image, thus leading to voluntary self- isolation. FM68

paralysis and skin pigmentation had shown up. I felt that time that they didn't like to get nearer to me so I decided that I'd just be the one to stay away and leave our place...) 68 P4: L4-11	
Oo. Sauna gud nga kuyug pa mi sa akung pamilya malipayun kayu mi pero pagkasakit nako kay nausab naman ilang pagtakad. *(Yes, I and my family used to be very happy but when I got sick their treatment towards me has changed...) 69 P4: L11-13*	One's condition has changed and disturbed family relationships. FM69
Nahadluk kayu sila sa akung sakit. Mahadluk kaayu sila muduol naku. *(They got really scared about my illness. They were very scared of approaching me. . .) 70 P4: L13-14*	The participant has felt the society's dread and fear about his disease. FM70
Nawagtangan ko ug paglaum sa didtu pa ko sa Manila kay	Efficient institutional support of services and care provides

wala may kausaban nako didtu. Karun sa pag balhin naku diri sa Cebu murag nibalik akung pagtuo nga mayu pa ko kay dinhi man ko hingpit na naulian. *(I lost my hope for some time when I was in Manila because there were no changes in me. But now that I transferred here in Cebu my hopes seem getting back becauseit' s here where I've really recovered.) 71 P4: 16-19*	the participant a beam of hope and a sheer of delight, reversing the despair once felt during the onset of his illness. FM71
Oo. Kay 1995 niuli man ko para mubisita murag lain na kayu amung mga tao didtu sa amu kay lain na ug tinagdan nako. *(Yes, the people in my place had treated me differently when I went home to visit my family in Leyte last 1995. . .) 72 P4: L21-23*	One's disease has impact on the way societal people would treat the stigmatized. FM72
Nag-una ilang huna-huna. Mahadlok sila na matakdan naku. *(They were thinking*	Participant has perceived societal fear of one's disease. FM73

ahead. They're scared that I might pass unto them my illness. . .) 73 P4: L23-24	
Lainan sila muduol naku. *(They don't like to get near me. . .) 74 P4: L24-25*	He feels being rebuffed and neglected due to fear of contracting the disease. FM74
Ako na lang gidawat ang ilang pag tratar nila diri naku bisag sakit para nako. *(I just accepted how they treated me even if it's painful for me. . .) 75 P4: L25-26*	Participant is left out with only one option to cope up and that's through acceptance. FM75
Nakababag ni sya sa akung pag skwela. *(It became a hindrance in my education. . .)* Tungod sa akung sakit wala ko'y nga skwela. *(Because of my illness I did not have a proper education. . .)* Ganahan unta ko mag teacher. *(I would like to become a teacher. . .) 76 P4: L28-30*	One's illness has put a barrier on the realization of one's potential and ambitions in life. FM 76
Ang akong giatubang karun ka yang akong sakit ni kumplekado sa akung atay.	He is worried about the prognosis of one's own illness; he is anxious about

Mao jud na akung kagul-an kung maka huna-huna ko sa akung sakit. *(What I am facing now is that my illness has complicate my liver. That's what I am really worried about everytime I think about my illness. . .) 77 P4: L33-36*	future health condition. Thinking on one's disease elicits fear. FM77
Okay ra man nako kay sa kadugay nakung pagtambal dinhi naulian man ko sa uban nakong mga sakit . kini lang jud ang sangla ang dugay mauli_i.*("It's okay for me somehow I've been healed from my other illness. It's only the leprosy that took time to be cured.") 78 P1: L5-8*	His faith, beliefs and hope have been restored and positive results have come . This directly translates into satisfaction of services rendered by the Leprosarium. This is the patient's affirmation of trust. Not only the institution of medicine and his particular treatment but to his own personal feelings about the illness and its ability to be cured. FM78

Wala ko'y mga pagbasul. *("I don't have any regrets.")* 79 P1: L8	The participant remains positive all throughout. FM79
Luya na akung lawas. Mulihay na naku ang akung kaubandiri naku tungod sa akung sakit. *("I feel weak... my colleagues become distance from me due to my condition.")* 80 P1: L9-10	The stigmatized individual is one who is not accepted and not accorded the respect, rights and regards of his peers, one who is disqualified from full social acceptance. FM80
Gidala ko nila sa San Lazaro para patambalan. Gi.ingnan ko sa akung amu ra mapauli na lang. gi tagaan ra ko sa sweldu unya gipauli sa tacloban.*("They brought me to san lazaro for treatment. My imloyer advised me to just go home. They gave me my salary and sent me back to tacloban.")* 81 P1: L14-16	It shows that his employer does not care about the health and welfare of his staff. The pacifying of the employees problem is common place. FM81

Wala ko nila taga-i ug kwarta parapatambal. Nay taga health center ni ingun naku na anhi diri sa cebu patambal.*("They did'nt give me money for treatment. A health worker advised me to come to Cebu for the treatment.")82 P1:L16-17*	Advocating the participant for a better treatment of his illness is crucial. FM82
Nakig buwag man naku akung asawa tungud sa akung sakit. wala sad ko nila bisitaha diri bisag kaisa. *("My wife broke up with me because of my illness. They never visited me her even once.")83 P1:L20-25*	Wife of the participant could not accept his illness and found it hard to put up of the condition towards the stigmatized individual.FM83
Wala naku'y planu na mabalik sa akung pamilya. Malipayun na man sad ko nagpuyu dinhi. *("I don't have plans of going back to my family. Anyhow I am already happy living here.")84 P1:L25-27*	The participant shows self-trust that he will be doing great even without going back to his family. As he also finds the belongingness from his new environment. FM84

Mahadluk sila naku ug mulikay na sila naku. Mao nga dili na lang ko mugawas. Nilakaw ko dayun sa amung lugar para maanhi sa cebu sa pagtambal. *("They become scared and avoid me. That is why I don't go out in my house anymore. I left our place and come to cebu right away for treatment.")85 P1:L28-31*	Social inequality and motive for negative community behavior are mostly found in the fact that people fear infection by germs. The extent of acceptance of deformed patience varied significantlyamong those among those facing and not facing problems due to their deformity. FM85
Malipay sad ko na nianhi . wala na may mahadluk naku dinhi kay pulus man mi parehas ug sakit.*("I am happy that I came here. No one is scared of me anymore because we are all in the same condition.")86 P1:L31-32*	Reducing stigma and increasingacceptance of leprosy-affected person will help in promoting favourable attitude towards leprosy. FM86

Dli nalang ko magpaduol nila. Ako na ln gang mo pa layo nila kay basig matakdan sila. *("I don't get near from them. I just try to stay away so that they will not be affected.")*87 P1:L35-36	Participant has created a zone for avoiding himself from the public hence for fear of spreading the disease. FM87
Gidawat na lng naku na mulikay naku ang mga tao mulikay naku tungud sa akung sakit . *("I have accepted that people will avoid me because of my illness.")*88 P1:L36-37	The stigmatized individual has accepted himself and the societal prejudice. FM88
Oo, kay tungud ani wala ko naka supurta sa akung pamilya . nawala akung trabahu.*("Yes, because of this I did not able to support my family. I lost my job.")*89 P1:L39-41	It limits or prevents them from fulfilling their normal roles in society. They may lose their economic independence as a results of losing their job, their physical independence as a result of disabilities. FM89
Naguol unta pero wala ko na lang huna-hunaa ako nalng gidawat akung sitwasyun.*("It*	The participant diverts his way of thinking in order for him not create ill-feeling, but

made me sad but I just I don't think about it anymore. I already accepted my situation.") *90 P1:L42-43*	to rather accept his condition. FM90
Wala man ko mawad-i ug pag-asa wala man mi'y problema sa pag puyu dinhi. *(" I did not lost my hope. We don'nt have problems living here.")91* *P1:L49-50*	The participant has a positive feeling and chooses to live with his life in normal way.FM91
Ako nalang gisalig sa ginoo tanan. Nagampo na lang sa tagaan ko ug taas na kinabuhi.*("I just trust everything to the lord. I just pray to have a longer life.")92* *P1:L50-52*	He strengthens his spiritual being. FM92

Wala sad ko maghuna-huna ana. Kini sakit gyud ni naku. Dili silut naku. *("I never think about it. This is really my desease. Not a punishment.")*	Misconception and negative attitude towards leprosy patient are prevalent on most community. FM93

Development of Cluster Themes and Emergent Themes

FORMULATED MEANINGS	CLUSTER THEMES	EMERGENT THEMES
*14 He has regrets though. He's of remorse because due to his physical condition, his family, friends and relatives almost forget and take him for granted completely.***36** Unexpected disease recognition and identification entails phase of depression. A feeling of	Regrets and Depression	"I Was Vanished Away Of Happiness": Negative Emotional Response

extreme sadness and denial were felt by the participant at first. ***50** The participant has regrets over some situations in the past.		
*19 He's not comfortable to live outside because the world inflicts pain and tears on his part that leads to lack of emotional security. ***70** The participant has felt the society's dread and fear about his disease. ***72** One's disease has impact on the way societal people would treat the stigmatized.***80**The stigmatized individual is one who is not accepted and not accorded the respect, rights and regards of his peers, one who is disqualified from full social acceptance. ***81**It shows that his employer does not	Societal Fear	

care about the health and welfare of his staff. The pacifying of the employees problem is common place.*85Social inequality and motive for negative community behavior are mostly found in the fact that people fear infection by germs. The extent of acceptance ofdeformed patience varied significantlyamong those among those facing and not facing problems due to their deformity.		
*20 He wants to convey to the public that leprosy has its own treatment and that it's not something to be scared of. *41 It is known to the participant that society is afraid of socializing and dealing with him especially when it involves skin-to-	Societal Perception	

skin or direct contact for fear of contracting the disease. It then eventually leads to participant's shame and low self- esteem. However he wants to inform the public that leprosy has its own treatment and once the Multi-drug Therapy (MDT) is initiated, it'd no longer be transmissible. ***53** Participant is a bit anxious of the society's perception of the disease. However, he is aware of the nature of the disease specifically its transmission. ***61** Participant manifests anxiety on how other people will react to his changes in physical appearance. ***64** Participant thinks other people have negative speculations about them after contracting the		

disease.		
*8 One's disease (leprosy) hinders realization of goals and dreams in life including stabilization of relationships among families, friends and relatives. ***29** The participant perceives leprosy as a physical and social barrier to attaining goals in life. Leprosy is thought to deter one's talents and potential. ***40** One's disease (Leprosy) limits one's capacity to attain goals, yearnings and dreams in life. ***57** Leprosy has been a hindrance to one's dreams and goals in life. There is a remorse over his present condition because it limits his former capability to attain those goals. ***65** Because of leprosy, he considers his	Hindrance	

dreams to be barred due to the physical and social limitation the disease brings. He undergoes the phase of bargaining. ***89**It limits or prevent them from fulfilling their normal roles in society. They may lose their economic independence as a results of losing their job, their physical independence as a result of disabilities.		
*13 Leaving behind their lives in the past is one of their ways to live and start something new. They no longer want to go back to the past experiences for the second time around. They only want to move forward. ***16** He views past as something different. He's a lot more hopeful with the present. ***49** Has a strong	Hope	"That Time Before Is Different, That of Today Is Better:"Positive Emotional Response

faith which keeps him to remain positive and hopeful in life. * **78**His faith, beliefs and hope have been restored and positive results have come . This directly translates into satisfaction of services rendered by the Leprosarium. This is the patient's affirmation of trust. Not only the institution of medicine and his particular treatment but to his own personal feelings about the illness and its ability to be cured.***79**The patient remains positive all throughout. ***84**The patient shows self-trust of himself that he will be doing great even without going back to his family. As he also find the belongingness from his new environment.***91** The		

participant has a positive feeling and chooses to live with his life in normal way. ***92**He strengthens his spiritual being.		
*37 There is a strong determination to recover soon completely especially that of the changes in physical appearance. ***38**One of the main reasons of wishing to get cured is about restoring back their previous functions for productivity.***45**There is a strong desire to get completely cured or healed.***52**Participant is aware of the nature of the Multi- Drug Therapy (MDT).***58**To get cured and recover soon are two yearnings which the participant wishes. Moreover, he still misses his	Determination to Recover	

family so much and is longing to see them someday. ***82**Facilitation the patience for a better treatment of his illness is crucial		
*43 There is acceptance by the family somehow.***47**There is a need for acceptance of one's condition.***75**Participant is left out with only one option to cope up and that's through acceptance. ***86**Reducing stigma and increasing acceptance of leprosy affected person will help in promoting favourable attitude towards leprosy. ***88**The stigmatized individual has accepted himself and the societal prejudice.	Acceptance	
*1 Disappointment and acceptance are two vital	Support	Live For Good Or Tramp For

stages of disease recognition and acquisition. Disappointment of one's self comes first accompanied by a lowering self- esteem due to a recognition of unpredictable disease or challenge in life. However, a good social support can aid in leading towards self-acceptance. For leprosy patients, their low self-esteem makes them think they are isolated from the rest of the world. However, when they are together alike having the same condition and living in the same environment, renewal of self- confidence will be gained. Togetherness, likeness and peer relation are all important. *2 Social support boosts self-security. *12 Institutional		Life

(Leprosarium) support and services facilitate feeling of security and help establish self- worth. The lepers are, however, contented and feel blessed to live in a non-discriminating environment that nurtures remaining potential and state of wellbeing. ***18** He assumes his co-leper to be his peers which he also considers his family. A bond between them is created through their likeness and togetherness being patients with the same condition and almost the same physical manifestations. ***21** The patients feel secured inside the leprosarium with the services and care rendered by the institution. The leprosarium becomes their safe haven to live peacefully.

They thought, had they not been brought there, living in the outside world would be more difficult.		
*17He's willing to go home if there's any chance, but is only limited to visiting his family and not to live there forever. He'd prefer and is more comfortable to stay inside the Leprosarium for good.*30He is happy to be in the Leprosarium. *32He likes to stay inside and if ever he gets well, he'd prefer to stay in the cottage than living in the outside world. He feels more safe and secured when living inside the leprosarium.	Staying Inside	
*3Low sense of self- worth and esteem is precipitated by the society's rebuff and prejudgments brought about by fear and	Self- isolation	Touch Me Not: Way Of Isolation And Disconnection

perception. It then becomes social stigma which makes the leper feel alone, peculiar and isolated.*9Changes in physical appearance among leprosy patients influence how people look at them and in return affect their perception of self- image. So they are afraid of going out where most of their physical image is exposed and becomes a subject for societal judgment and for fear of being humiliated.*11They are forced to move out of the house for fear of transmitting the disease to other family members and infecting those whom he loves. *25Discrimination is common. It tortures them verbally.*26He thinks his disease becomes something		

to be scared of that's why others would avoid him.***31**He prefers not to go outside to avoid encountering obvious signs of discrimination.***39**Exposure to the society is avoided due to perception of shame brought about by one's disturbed self- image.***42** Hiding from the society is their way of controlling or avoiding getting hurt.***62** Because of awareness on societal stigma, lepers tend to hide from the society in order to isolate themselves in a way they are less-threatened by discrimination. ***87**Patient has created his zone of avoiding himself from the public hence for fear of spreading the disease. FM87		

*5 Suppression and repression are used as coping mechanisms to forget or put into the subconscious mind those hurtful words or any unpleasant experience before. This is to lessen or stop adding burden of pain, worries and guilt inside.***6**Acceptance comes and is aided to happen when one's own anxiety is displaced and released through outside physical activity. Activities such as recreation and amusement maintains lepers' sense of physical function and emotional satisfaction.***22**They feel taken for granted and forgotten by their families but they repressed it in	Psychological Conditioning	

their subconscious minds so as not to add emotional guilt and feelings of hopelessness. An activity for diversion becomes their way of mitigating the despair inside them and the emotional stress brought by the idea that they're forsaken not just by their families but by the society in general.**27**He has accepted himself and his disease so he shrugs at other people's prejudice.**28**He is indifferent to what others might say about his disease/ condition. Minding about their statements might only precipitate self- pity and elicit both emotional and psychological jeopardy.**35**Aware of the society's prejudice and discrimination but is willing		

to pay no attention to them because of self-acceptance.**54**Tolerating what others say is a coping strategy to avoid disappointment.**56**The participant is willing to tolerate discrimination from the society because he perceived leprosy as uncontrollable, something he never wished to have and whose reason of having is not known to him.**59**He relates psychological mind set as a determinant to one's own physical condition. Thinking positively, for him, helps avoid his disease from getting worse.**90**The patient diverts his way of thinking in order for him not create ill-feeling, that that he just accepts his		

condition.		
*7 He conceives leprosy to be caused by physiologic insufficiencies and lack of optimum health habits related to work and stress of his previous job. Specifically, he attributed inadequate rest as one of the major determinants of developing leprosy.***15**He perceived his disease to be caused by external factors such as occupation, inadequate rest and companion. He does not believe that it comes from internal factors such as a person's attitude and character attributed to one's own personality in general. ***24**He attributed the predisposing factors of his disease to include inadequate rest due to his	External Factor	A Struggle For Mammon, A Battle For One's Soul

previous job.***33**He lacks enough knowledge about the aetiology of the disease. ***48**For him, leprosy is caused by external factors such as work- related stress and inadequate rest.***51**One of the perceived reasons for having leprosy is work-related factor.		
*34 Does not attribute one's disease as God's plan. He isn't certain with what really causes the disease. ***44**Does not attribute one's disease to be God's plan. Each one of us has our own share of sins.***60**The participant does not perceive the relationship between attitude and one's own illness. ***66**The participant also wonders whether his condition is a punishment. Accepting it	Internal Factor	

becomes his coping strategy to move forward. Nonetheless, he is uncertain whether he can still go back to his normal life or not after overcoming the challenge wrought by his condition.		
*4 Lepers try to remain intact and linked with the outside world especially to their families and nearest kin, no matter how they're being forsaken and taken for granted. They still long to see their families well and in good condition.*10Relationship changes and the role-pattern is disturbed between the family members and the patient after recognition of disease condition. *63For him, his 007Afamily becomes his	Family	Relationship and Society

motivation to recover soon.***67**Family. They are the sole motivation for the patient to recover. He becomes hopeful because of them.***69**One's condition has changed and disturbed family relationships. ***83**Wife of the patient could not accept his illness and found it hard to put up of the condition towards to the stigmatized individual.		
*23They are yearning to be loved and to feel the sense of belongingness, that somehow they are given worth and importance by the society and the world outside.***55**Participant wants to reconcile with the society and foster humane relationship.	Reconciliation with the Society	

BIBLIOGRAPHY

Insert cha **Journals**

Abedi, Heidarali et al. (2013). An Exploration of Health, Family and Economic Experiences of Leprosy Patients, Iran. *Pakistan Journal of   Biological Sciences, 16: 927-932*

Girao, Régio José Santiago et al. (2013).Leprosy Teatment Drop- out: A   Systematic   Review. International Archives of Medicine. 6:34

Heijnders, M. L. (2004). Experiencing Leprosy: Perceiving and Coping with   Leprosy and its Treatment. *Lep Review .* (2004) 75: 327-337

Joseph, G. A. & Rao, P. S. (1999). Impact of Leprosy on Quality of Life. *Bulletin   of the World Health Organization.* 77(6):515-7

Kazeem, Omobolanle & Abegun, Temitayo. (2011). Leprosy Stigma:Ironing Out   the Creases. *Lepra Health in Action.* (2011) 82: 103-108

Kumar A., Anbalagan M. (1983). Socio- economic Experiences of Leprosy Patients.   *U.S. National Library of Medicine.*55(2):314-21

Luka, Edward Eremugo . (2012). Understanding the Stigma of Leprosy. South   Sudan Medical Journal

Mankar, Madhavi J., Joshi, Sumedha M., Velankar, Deepa H., et al.(2011). A   Comparative Study of the Quality of Life, Knowledge, Attitude and Belief   About Leprosy Disease Among Leprosy Patients and Community Members   in   Shantivan   Leprosy Rehabilitation C entre, Nere, Maharashtra, *India.*
     *Journal of Global Infectious Diseases .***3**(4): 378–382

 Mishra C.P. & Gupta, M. K. (2010). Editorial: Leprosy and Stigma. *Indian J Prev   Soc. Med.*41: 1(2)

Peters, Ruth M.H et al. (2013). The Meaning of Leprosy and

Everyday   Experiences: An Exploration in Cirebon, Indonesia.

Journal of Tropical   Medicine

Rafferty, J., 2005. Curing the stigma of leprosy. Lepr. Rev., 76: 119-126.

Shosha, Ghada Abhu. (2012). Employment of Colaizzi's Strategy in Descriptive   Phenomenology: Reflection of a Researcher. *European Scientific Journal.*   (8) 27: 33-34

Shumen, Chen et al. (2005). Qualitative assessment of social, economic and medical needs for ex-leprosy patients living in leprosy villages in   Shandong Province, The People's Republic of China. *Lepr Rev.* 76, 335–   347

Van Brakel, Wim H. (2003). Measuring Leprosy Stigma- a Preliminary Review   of the Leprsosy Literature. *International Journal of Leprosy and Other Mycobacterial Diseases.* 71 (3): 190-197

Electronic and Internet Sources

Crisostomo, Sheila. (2013). Phl accounts for big number of leprosy cases in   W. Pacific. *The Philippine Star.*
      <http://www.philstar.com/science-and   t
      echnology/2013/02/28/913858/phl-accounts-big-number-leprosy-cases- w.-pacific>

http://www.ilep.org.uk/ilep-co-ordination/leprosy-around-the-world/asia/philippines/

International Archives of Medicine. (2013).   Leprosy   Treatment Drop-out: A   Systematic Review.

Journal of Tropical Medicine. (2013). The Meaning of Leprosy and Everyday   Experiences: An Exploration in Cirebon, Indonesia.

      <http://www.hindawi.com/journals/jtm/2013/507034/>

Smith,   Darvin   Scott.   (2014).Leprosy.   MedSCape
      <http://emedicine.medscape.com/article/220455-overview
≥

South Sudan Medical Journal. (2012). Understanding the Stigma of Leprosy.
      <http://www.southsudanmedicaljournal.com/archive/augu
st-   2010/understanding-the-stigma-of-leprosy.html>

World   Health   Organization.   (2014).   Prevalence   of   Leprosy.
      http://www.who.int/lep/situation/prevalence/en/

ABOUT THE AUTHOR

The author is a Philippine Registered Nurse. He had earned his Bachelor of Science in Nursing with Latin Honors 'Cum Laude' in March 2015. He also graduated High School Valedictorian way back in year 2011. He was a recipient of St. Brother Benilde Medal of Academic Excellence and many other awards bestowed after his steadfast dedication and love for Science and Literature. He had been a Student Editor for several years and a writer by blood. Presently, he is a Licensed Financial Advisor / Investment Planner and a Publishing Consultant.

The main impetus for his desire to understand the lived experiences of a leper was triggered by his curiosity on how a leprosarium exactly looks like. Putting himself in the shoe of ostracism allows him to fathomize the real cause of social stigma and uncover leper's stories never made known or told before.

www.ingramcontent.com/pod-product-compliance
Lightning Source LLC
Chambersburg PA
CBHW071305220526
45468CB00001B/277